Anything Can Be Healed

"Shared in a down-to-earth style that everyone can digest, *Anything Can Be Healed* shows the extraordinary depths of consciousness that can be accessed by anyone wishing to heal or be healed. Healing isn't rocket science, and when approached in a certain way, miracles do happen. This book demonstrates exactly how to create rapid, effective change in one's own or another's reality, instigating powerful healing."

JERRY SARGEANT
founder of Star Magic Healing and author of
Star Magic: Heal the You-Niverse

"As one who recognizes the importance of personal responsibility for one's own healing and experiences, I found *Anything Can Be Healed* a hugely valuable book, full of healer wisdom, depth, and integrity from start to finish. There is insight here for novices and advanced healers alike, with informative chakra reference charts. Recognizing the divine and the healing potential in all of us, Martin offers healing techniques and insights into personal empowerment and sovereignty over our own healing, life, and experiences."

NIKKI GRESHAM-RECORD
psychologist, energy healer, and author of
Working with Chakras for Belief Change: The Healing InSight Method

Anything
Can Be Healed

The Body Mirror System
of Healing with Chakras

MARTIN BROFMAN

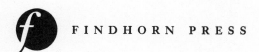

FINDHORN PRESS

Findhorn Press
One Park Street
Rochester, Vermont 05767
www.findhornpress.com

Findhorn Press is a division of Inner Traditions International

Disclaimer
The information in this book is given in good faith and is neither intended to diagnose any physical or mental condition nor to serve as a substitute for informed medical advice or care. Please contact your health professional for medical advice and treatment. Neither author nor publisher can be held liable by any person for any loss or damage whatsoever which may arise from the use of this book or any of the information therein.

Cataloging-in-Publication data for this title is available from the Library of Congress

ISBN 978-1-62055-896-6 (print)
ISBN 978-1-62055-897-3 (ebook)

Printed and bound in the United States

10 9 8 7 6 5 4 3

Edited by Lynn Barton
Text design and layout by Geoff Green Book Design CB24 4GL
This book was typeset in Kingfisher
Artwork by Nathalie Huguet, except for pp. 58, 63, 104, 157 (top two), 160, 161, 163, 212 (bottom two) by Hélène Dubois; p.128 by Richard Crookes

To send correspondence to the author of this book, mail a first-class letter to Annick Brofman c/o Inner Traditions • Bear & Company, One Park Street, Rochester, VT 05767, USA and we will forward the communication, or contact the Brofman Foundation directly at **https://brofman -foundation.org** or **angel@healer.ch**

To my Spirit,
who volunteered for this assignment,
and continues to guide me to its
ongoing unfolding and fruition.

Contents

Foreword
by Anna Parkinson

Martin Brofman was a powerful being who changed the course of many lives. My first meeting with him certainly changed mine. It was quite unexpected. I had an inoperable brain tumor and though I had explored all the medical avenues for dealing with it, I was getting nowhere and going around in circles. After many weeks of hesitation, of listening to Martin's talks and learning his story, I felt compelled to overcome my resistance and go to ask Martin for healing.

The experience was a revelation, not simply because of the palpable energy that transmits when one person wishes to heal another, but because Martin had the ability to explain what was happening in a way I could understand. Almost immediately afterwards, disparate strands of my life clicked into place in an entirely comprehensible and logical relationship. I discovered a new perspective, and with it, a new sense of ownership of my body and the life I chose to live. Martin opened my eyes to the way my inner world expresses itself through my body and what happens in my life. This is the substance of the ideas he explains in this book. This is the journey you have in store from reading and practicing the techniques he perfected. Your inner world, moreover, connects you to a much deeper sense of your self and your purpose than you may be familiar with. In this way, your body can be your guide to a more fulfilling and happier life.

In his preface to this book, Martin says he didn't believe in any of the ideas explained in this book before 1975. It was his body that faced him with a life-threatening situation he was forced to find a way out of. When the medical profession couldn't help, he had to dig deep into the wisdom of ancient ideas about the relationship of his invisible consciousness to his physical body to find another way to live. It was do or die. This was exactly the path that led me to Martin's door more than a quarter of a century later. I was a broadcast journalist for BBC current affairs and accustomed to assessing truth by measurable facts. This had made me underestimate the power of the unmeasurable or invisible, of emotional truth in myself and others, and overestimate the validity of appearances.

As the psychologist William James pointed out we tend to forget that we are all, after all, "invisible." The great motivating factors of our lives are undetectable to our normal sense of vision. Neither love, desire, passion, envy, nor anger can be seen, but they are all potent energies, which create tangible physical changes in our lives. As we all know, and as the writer William Bruce Cameron said, "Not everything that counts can be counted and not everything that can be counted counts."

The invisible and the uncountable is so frustrating to the scientific method that has produced the modern environment for most of us that it tends to be dismissed. In so doing, this kind of thinking makes a basic mistake. It is like looking at a box and dismissing the space within it, because there is nothing visible or countable there. The space within is, however, the point of the box.

In a similar way, modern medicine tends to treat people as mechanical beings, assessing our health, happiness, and future by the physical aspects of our bodies and attempting to modify anything irregular with drugs that have a contrary physical effect. Most of us have experienced that this doesn't always work. The same drug has different effects on different people. Because of course although human bodies function normally in the same way, no two individuals have exactly the same emotional experience.

Martin's approach is apparently simple. A happy person is a healthy person. When you are happy, your body functions in perfect harmony and balance. When you are unhappy, the tension in your body will help you to understand emotional tensions you may not have been conscious of. This is the essence of ancient philosophies that accept the perfect design and functioning of natural organisms as beyond human conception. The Buddha is reputed to have said, "There is no way to happiness. Happiness is the way." Anyone who has tried to focus on this goal will find it contains enough challenges to occupy a whole lifetime as well as inconceivable joys and unimaginable triumphs.

It would be a mistake, however, to confuse apparent simplicity with lack of logic. Martin's genius was to focus his intelligence on anything that appeared hazy or illogical and ask questions, while at the same time entertaining the perspective that human beings form part of a greater evolutionary truth that has not been measured by scientific methods but perceived and described by spiritual ones. The chain of reaction that emotions set up in our bodies is highly logical, and Martin has shown how it can be understood like any logical language. Of course, this would be meaningless if it could not be understood by the person who needs healing. But, after decades of applying this method in healing hundreds of people, Martin's experience was that this body language is understood by the person who needs healing. Once understood, the mystery to behold is how physical changes follow. It is as though the body is holding on to the truth until the person inside the body gets it.

My physical symptoms did not disappear immediately after I met Martin, but his teaching and the Body Mirror Healing System he devised, which you find explained in this book, provided a clear pathway to show how physical symptoms can disappear. Martin's constant message was to take charge of creating the life you want to lead: to be the director of your own movie, as he often put it. The only limitations are the ones we place on ourselves, and the power our minds can access is limitless.

Not knowing what I would find at the end of the path, drawn on by curiosity, I set about learning as much about healing as I could. I discovered, to my astonishment, that I had the ability to heal others, and that, with patient and persistent work on myself, my own symptoms diminished until, eventually, the tumor itself disappeared. I did not always believe in the end result I would achieve, but I allowed myself to imagine it, with greater and greater confidence. I have Martin and the Body Mirror Healing method to thank for that. In the years since, I have found that healing is constantly teaching me, adding new dimensions to my experience that I could never have arrived at by logical means but which have power because they are true, for me and for you.

Martin's vision of the power of healing delivered a method, Body Mirror Healing, that he was motivated to share, and he devoted his life to teaching it all around the world. He maintained that children could learn it in as little as two days and that the practice of healing itself would teach them what they needed to know. That has certainly been my experience. The practice of healing, oneself or others, is a great teacher.

While the wisdom of ancient shamans and philosophers has often been used to exert power over other people, Martin's genius was to open our eyes to the power within us all. He was a stickler for detail, and he could be exacting, but he was infinitely generous in his perception of superhuman power in every individual. He never ceased to remind people to expand their notions of what is possible. "Whatever one human being can do, you can do too." The first time I met him his parting shot was along those lines. "People think you are odd if you say, 'I am Divine,' but it's true," he said. "The power of divine energy is in us all." I understood at once. "It's like a verb you learn at school," I replied. "I am divine, you are divine, he, she, it is divine…" He nodded enthusiastically.

Whatever your motivation for picking up this book, whatever you hope to find in it, persevere with the ideas it contains and put them to the test.

You will find your world expanding in delightful and surprising ways, for your own benefit and for those around you. With an open heart and mind, I trust you will discover how "Anything can be healed."

ANNA PARKINSON

Author of *Change Your Mind, Heal Your Body*

Carlisle, 28th November 2018

Preface

Before 1975, I didn't believe in any of the ideas contained in this book. It was only because I was diagnosed as being terminally ill with a tumor in my spinal cord and given one or two months to live that I was stimulated to research the relationship between my consciousness and my body in order to heal myself.

I decided to work on myself, using techniques of relaxation, visualization, positive thinking, meditation, and affirmations that I had learned through a program called the Silva Method. During this time, motivated by the need to heal myself, I also explored Eastern religions and esoteric philosophies, and Western psychology, as well, searching in every area that could provide any information I could use to save my life.

After two months of working on myself, I was rewarded by hearing the doctors declare that they must have made a mistake. There was no longer a tumor, or any symptoms.

When my own healing was complete, I began teaching others the self-healing tools I had used, sharing the insights I had gained during my own process. Some of those who came to me asked me to heal them. I was reluctant at first, feeling that each of us has the power and the ability to heal ourselves. Some people, however, had a difficult time accepting that, or did not know how to generate for themselves the degree of clarity and objectivity necessary for the process. They believed more in my ability to heal them than in their ability to heal themselves. No matter how much I insisted that they could do it themselves, they held their perception that I should be the one to do it for them. If I refused, they left without being healed, and I did not feel good with that.

I thought that if I were writing the script to this scenario, I could have done a better job, seeing an ending in which the people were healed when they left, so I agreed to participate in the role of healer in their process. As I worked with more and more people, I could see more and more the relationship between what was happening in their bodies and what was happening in their consciousnesses. Gradually, a model developed which seemed to contain all the ideas I had explored, and which also reflected my experiences, as well as what I had seen in the healings in which I had participated. The model developed into a system of healing that I decided to call the Body Mirror System, to represent the idea that one's body is a mirror of one's life.

When healing is needed, the parts of our body that do not work well reflect the parts of our life that do not work well, that is, the parts of our life about which there is stress and tension in our consciousness. The stress in our consciousness about a particular part of our life is stored as tension on the physical level in a particular part of our body. Thus, the body can be seen as a map of the consciousness. The healing process involves releasing the tensions not only from the body but also from the consciousness, returning to our natural state of balance.

Healing, since it has existed as a concept, has often been seen with misunderstanding, suspicion, and awe. Society has always considered the process as something extraordinary and mysterious, and only accessible to shamans, medicine men, those with special gifts or a direct telephone connection with God, or some other condition not normally associated with ordinary people when, in fact, we all have these gifts, and we are all healers.

The purpose of this book is to present healing as a technology of consciousness, that is, a set of tools that is accessible to anyone who wishes to learn the process. It is a technical manual of the healing process, combining concepts found in Eastern traditions with those in Western psychology. Readers who are familiar with esoteric philosophies will find a clarification of concepts, while those who do not have any background in these areas will find the ideas and techniques so simply presented that they will be able to grasp them easily and thus apply them just as easily.

This book contains the ideas, principles, and philosophies that make up the Body Mirror System of Healing and Self-Knowledge. May it help you to know yourself, and to know how to heal yourself and others.

No illness exists that someone, somewhere, has not been healed of.

What one person can do, any person can do.

Anything can be healed.

Orientation

Introduction

Everything begins in your consciousness.

Everything that happens in your life, and everything that happens in your body, begins with something happening in your own consciousness.

As you are presented with conditions in your life, you choose to respond in a particular way. You make decisions. You decide what to feel, what to think, what to do. Or you decide to not decide. That, too, is a decision that you take.

This process is not one that begins at a certain age. It is always true, and has always been true. It is true now. You have been doing this as a consciousness, as a spirit, from before the time you were born into a human body, through infancy, childhood, and adolescence, and you will continue to do so through your adult life, and even after you leave your human biological vehicle.

When you respond to conditions optimally, you remain in balance, and the process continues. When you respond in a way that results in tension or physical symptoms, it means that something is not successful, and has not been working well for you. Something is out of balance.

The natural state of your consciousness is balance. Healing is a return to your natural state of balance and wholeness. In our society, you have been taught to orient yourself toward the belief that the causes of illness or injury are outside yourself. While this is indeed true on the physical plane, it is also true that this only happens when the conditions in your consciousness permit it.

If you continue to orient yourself toward seeking outer cures, outer remedies, you tend to not see the conditions in your life and the tensions in your consciousness that correlate with and, in fact, create the symptoms on the physical level. You then see yourself as a victim of your environment. You also tend to not clear the tensions from your consciousness that stand between you and the health and happiness you seek.

If you choose to do something about the symptoms in a way that is different from the modern traditional approaches, you can start this process so by re-orienting yourself to the perception that everything begins in your own consciousness. In this way, you also take responsibility for everything that happens in your body, and in your life, and for what you choose to put or allow yourself to accept into your consciousness.

You are then able to remind yourself of the degree to which you create your reality. You can also remind yourself of your unlimited natural abilities, and of the natural inner tools you have always had for healing, and how to use them. You can also remember that you can choose to respond to your environment in a different way—one that works better for you.

This book is intended to be your reminder of the connections between your consciousness and your body. It is also a user's manual for the equipment you have had since you came into this world, as well as for the tools for working with it, which are always available to you, and to us all.

We are all healers, and somewhere deep inside we know that anything can be healed.

CHAPTER 1

Healers and Healing

We define healing as "returning to the experience of balance (harmony) and wellness." One who heals another is helping the other return to the experience of wellness. Those healing themselves, or involved in self-healing, are returning themselves to the experience of wellness.

The word *healing* is used to describe the process that has as its intention the return to wellness of the subject, the person receiving the healing. It is also the name we give to the end result when the process is successful. We say that the person has had a healing, and is healed.

The degree of success of the healing may be partial or total. When it is partial, the person has experienced some kind of improvement. We say that they have experienced a healing, with partial results (so far). When the effects are total, we say that the person has been healed.

A *healer* is someone participating in the process of healing, having the intention of helping the subject return to the experience of wellness. We also use the same name to describe someone who has had successful results in this role in the past. Since only healers can heal, anyone who has successfully performed a healing must be a healer.

What is implied is that those we call healers *have the ability* to have successful results with the process. We believe that everyone is born with this ability and only needs to learn how to use the tools they already have. To this degree, we believe that we are all healers, either latent or accomplished.

As with medicine, results of healings may not be guaranteed. When the process is successful, however, it is because of a combination of conditions that have been met, and which can be quantified. These include the degree of skill of the healer in using the tools available; the degree to which the one needing the healing is open to it, and to the process of change that necessarily accompanies it; and also the dynamics of interaction between the healer and the healee, the subject of the healing.

Obviously, many levels of healing are possible, including physical, mental, emotional, and spiritual, and also many categories of healers. Some healers work with energy from God and feel they are only channels for the work being done by God. Others work with more of a sense of personal involvement in the healing, feeling it is they who are doing something, and they may not even believe in God. Either way, people are being healed. There is no reason for anyone to continue to suffer if a means of relief is available, as a humanitarian gesture freely offered by someone with different beliefs and having the appropriate tools and skills.

Some healers work with ideas of maintaining the purity of the vehicle, their body, through which the healing energy must pass, and others work with the idea that the love that heals is pure, regardless of the individual fuel requirements or the condition of that vehicle. Some healers eat meat, while others are vegetarians.

Some shamanic techniques involve the use of drugs, while other healers avoid them. Some healers use substances, such as herbs and various kinds of medicines, while others work only with the power of consciousness. Some healers feel good to be around, while others are best loved from a distance. What all have in common is that they have the ability to help another being return to the experience of wholeness. They all serve the community around them by doing something that helps the members of that community.

When we consider all this, it is evident that there is no way that you must change your way of being in order to enter the community of healers. The first rule is just to be yourself and to do whatever works best for you, even if you do it differently from everyone else around you.

It doesn't matter what your personal habits are, your eating habits, sexual habits, or social skills. Your value to the community is your ability to heal others.

When you are successful with that, you are a healer, and that is something that can never be taken away from you, or invalidated by any other person, whatever their limiting ideas may be.

When functioning as a healer, you are a member of a community of healers that extends into every segment of our population, fitting in with the milieu in which it functions. Healers are in every part of society where healing is needed, and until now, no segment of our society has been exempt. Even healers sometimes need healing.

Some healers work in the scientific community, others in the spiritual community, the military, and in politics. Healers are found in the well-respected and socially acceptable circles of society, as well as in subcultures and countercultures.

Being able to use a set of tools effectively to heal another does not make one inherently more powerful or better than another, any more than knowing how to read makes one more powerful or better than another. Both are valuable skills that anyone can learn, and that are, in fact, taught to children. How can we inflate ourselves over our ability to use tools that can be learned by six-year-old children?

It is true that some healers may have preyed on the superstition and ignorance of those around them to advance their own private purposes. However, that is less and less common as more people discover just how accessible and easy is the ability to use the tools of healing, such as those presented in this book.

It's not a question of whether healing works, but rather one of how it works. This book is intended to explain how healing works.

Anyone can use these tools.

Anyone can heal.

Anything can be healed.

CHAPTER 2

Alternative Realities

To begin with, we must get away from the idea that there is only one way that things work, just one reality. We will explore here the idea of alternative realities in which things happen in different ways.

We are each a consciousness in a body. We each decide what to think and what to feel. We choose our perceptions, and our perceptions create our reality.

Our perceptions are the subjective way we interpret all of the information coming into our consciousness from the world around us.

It is as if there is a bubble around each of us. Some of the information coming through this bubble is filtered to the surface and presented to our conscious attention to be noticed. The rest does not register consciously, but travels through the bubble and is stored at deeper levels of our consciousness. Our ideas, beliefs, desires, and feelings color the bubble filtering our perceptions; so much so that people with different bubbles looking at the same thing can have totally different perceptions of what they are watching.

A person in a red bubble, for example, will see the world as red, while a person in a blue bubble will see it as blue, and we can imagine the conversation between these two discussing the color of the world. From a certain point of view, they are both correct about what they report, and all of their perceptions affirm their truth. Yet from another point of view, perhaps neither perception represents objective reality. Perhaps the world is neither red nor blue. All that we know to be true for sure is that one person sees it as red and another as blue, so we have a sense of the nature of each of the bubbles, each of the filters. In this way, we have a basis for communication and exchange of ideas.

While we each may see the same events in the outer world, our respective bubbles color our interpretation of these events. Looking at our interpretation can give us an idea of the nature of our own beliefs and perceptions, since it is these that "color" our bubbles. Someone believing that competition and conflict are universal will see only that, while someone else may just as clearly see that the world is full of people motivated by love and expressing it, and sometimes reacting to the perception that it is not there.

It is easy to see how our perceptions can then predispose us to acting in certain ways that not only play into the apparent scenario we perceive, but actually create and continue it. A man insecure about his lover, for example, can actually drive away that lover with his insecurities, justifying his perceptions, proving that he was right, yet at the same time, having created the scenario in the first place.

There's a story about a man whose car had a flat tire, not far from a farmhouse in a remote farming community. The man thought, "There's a farmhouse. I'm sure that they have tools that I can use to fix the flat tire."

As he walked toward the farmhouse, he thought, "It will be really helpful to me to use those tools. I can be generous, and give the farmer ten dollars to use the tools. I'm sure he will appreciate that."

As he walked farther, he thought, "This is really remote, and we're far from any other civilization. If that farmer wanted to charge me twenty-five dollars to use his tools, I would have to pay it."

Farther along, he thought, angrily, "We're really deserted here. If that farmer wanted to charge me fifty dollars to use his tools, I would have no choice but to pay it!"

By the time he reached the farmhouse, knocking on the door, he was really furious, and as the farmer opened the door, the man yelled at the farmer, "So, how much are you going to charge me to use your tools, you thief?"

So we can see how the man, predisposed to acting in certain ways, not only played into the apparent scenario he perceived, but actually created it.

When we talk about our perceptions creating our reality, we are talking not only of our perceptual filters, but also the way things happen. This means that even apparently physical cause-and-effect relationships are different in different realities, in different paradigms.

For example, those wanting to become thinner may believe that to do so, they must be aware of the calories they take in with their food compared to the calories they burn through their activities. If they take in more calories than they burn, they will put on weight, and if they burn more calories than they take in, they will become thinner. One way to become thinner, then, is to eat foods that provide fewer calories than is needed to consume them. Grapefruit is such a food. Within this reality, then, if we eat grapefruit, we can expect to become thinner.

Within a different reality, calories have little to do with weight, since calories are consumed immediately. We must be aware of carbohydrates since they are stored in the body as fat. If we want to become thinner, we must reduce our intake of carbohydrates. Since grapefruit, like all fruit, contains carbohydrates, within this reality, if we eat a lot of grapefruit, we will put on weight!

Both realities are true, and people believing in each reality can easily prove that they are both right. One reality does not preclude the other. One does not have to be wrong for the other to be right. Both are right, and yet things happen in different ways within each reality.

What will happen when you eat a grapefruit? Will you put on weight, or will you become thinner?

First, it depends on what you believe will happen when you eat the grapefruit. If you believe you will put on weight, you will. If you believe you will become thinner, you will. If you really don't know what will happen, you must eat the grapefruit to find out. Then you can identify with one reality or the other and know what is true for you. At the same time, you can now know that something else may be true for another person.

Whatever you believe to be true is true—for you!

Where do your beliefs come from?

When you are presented with another person's beliefs, you are free to accept them or reject them. If you choose to accept somebody else's beliefs as true for you as well, you then adopt them as yours. You can decide for yourself that since an expert says so, it must be true that eating grapefruit makes you thin. Or fat. As you decide.

Another way to create a belief in your own consciousness is to define it from the way you have interpreted your own experiences. You might start with no idea of what is true for you and no idea what to believe. You begin with an experience: you eat the grapefruit, not knowing what might happen.

Next, you examine the effects of the experience. You interpret your experience in a certain way, describing it to yourself with certain words. In doing so, you create a certain belief. You decide, for example, "Eating grapefruit makes me thin, because when I ate a lot of grapefruit, I became thinner."

The words that you use to describe your experience create your beliefs, and therefore your reality.

After your experiences have defined your beliefs, your beliefs define and create your experience, so that you will discover that whatever you believe to be true is true for you. You will attract to yourself, and will have more of a tendency to notice, those experiences that affirm your truth.

Thus, someone believing something different can have something different that is true for them. Also, by changing your beliefs, you can change the way things happen within your paradigm, within your reality. Thus, if something has been not working optimally for you, by exploring different beliefs, you can discover a way to have things work for you in a different way, the way you would like them to. You can find a way to achieve what you want.

Within a reality of the physical sciences, a person might be told that they have a grave illness for which nothing can be done. Within this reality, if nothing changes, they will certainly die. If they choose to explore alternative realities in which there is a way out of their condition, there is a chance that they can continue to live, in health and harmony.

When the healing happens, it may happen in a way that seems to suspend or violate certain physical laws of chemistry, biology, or physics. These laws, though, are not absolute dictates, but just attempts to predict behavior on the basis of past experience and empirical data. They are considered laws only until something happens that makes it necessary to consider additional factors, and modify these laws.

For example, if you throw something into the air, it comes down. No matter how many times you repeat the process, the result is the same. You can decide, as a law, that "What goes up must come down." This happens until you throw something with such force that it escapes the earth's gravity, and you are obliged to change the laws to consider other factors.

When we look at the paradigm of healing, even though it may seem that we are breaking the "laws" of biology, chemistry, and physics, no laws are actually being violated. It's just that other laws are being obeyed, since things happen in different ways within different realities.

Healing is presented, then, as an alternative bubble to the reality of the traditional medical sciences. Any bubble can be presented and look as if it is the only reality that exists. If we release the idea that there is only one reality, we can then consider alternative realities that can exist either alone or in combination with other realities.

Some people choose to combine the different realities, taking elements of each that work best for them. Others, who have been told by the traditional sciences that nothing can be done for them, might prefer to dedicate themselves totally to the alternative paradigms.

What is of primary importance is doing what works best for you, and not rejecting any idea or method that may help you in some way.

This handbook is the presentation of the truths, dynamics, and cause-and-effect relationships that exist within the bubble that represents the reality, the paradigm, of the Body Mirror System of Healing.

It does not invalidate any other realities, but simply provides an alternative. Within this reality, we hold the perception that anything can be healed.

CHAPTER 3

The Human Energy System

You are a consciousness. Consciousness can be defined as "the experience of being." You are therefore a being, experiencing being. You have always been that, and you will always be that. While in a human form, you call yourself a human being.

Consciousness can also be described as a form of energy. Sometimes it is known as "life energy." When consciousness, or life energy, leaves the body, the body dies. What we refer to as the physical body is not who you are, but rather, only a vehicle for the consciousness that you are. At the same time, it is an extension, a denser aspect, of your consciousness/ energy, and so it also reflects the conditions of the consciousness that you are.

Together, you and your body (bodies, if we include the subtle bodies) constitute an energy system, that is, different densities of energy, at different frequencies, in a dynamic relationship.

While such ideas have been known and communicated for thousands of years, not until recently has evidence of them been demonstrated scientifically. Now, however, through the process of Kirlian photography, this is possible, and has been done. With this system of photography, an electrical current is passed through a photographic plate while a picture is being taken of something in contact with the plate. At first, pictures were taken of leaves, and when the pictures were developed, the image of the physical leaf was surrounded by what appeared to be an energy field radiating from the physical leaf.

When a part of the leaf was cut away and another Kirlian photograph was taken, the image of the physical leaf was seen with the part cut away, but the energy field surrounding the physical leaf was whole, with no part cut away. It became evident that the energy field of the leaf was not just something radiating from the physical leaf, but rather had a separate existence from it.

When a Kirlian photograph is taken of someone's hand, there appears a pattern of energy. It has been demonstrated that healers who have had Kirlian photographs taken of their hands have been able to influence the pattern of energy, so that when they consciously sent energy through their hands, the pattern shown on the Kirlian photograph changed.

The Kirlian photographs, then, are not reflecting the physical structure of the hand, but rather the consciousness and energy field of the person whose hand it is. A change in the consciousness of the person is reflected in the Kirlian photographs as a change in the person's energy field.

Practitioners of Kirlian photography have been able to quantify the energy field thus shown, to identify "weak spots" in the person's energy field, which correlate with particular physical weaknesses, or symptoms. In fact, the weaknesses in the energy field can be detected even before there is any evidence of the weaknesses on the physical level.

A change in consciousness creates a change in the energy field. A change in the energy field appears before there is a change on the physical level. Thus, there is a direction of manifestation, from consciousness, to the energy field, to the physical body.

Consciousness —> Energy Field —> Physical Body

When we look at the process in this way, it becomes clear that it is not the physical body that creates the energy field, but rather, the energy field, the effect of the consciousness, that creates the physical body.

What we see as the physical body is the end result of a process that begins with the consciousness. The consciousness, the energy field, and the physical body are all in a state of balance relative to each other. When there is a sufficient change in the consciousness caused by a decision or reaction creating tension, the energy field and the physical body will come into balance with it, and the symptom will appear as tension in the body, reflecting the tension in the consciousness.

During a healing, when the energy field is being repaired and rebalanced, the consciousness and the physical body will come into a new state of balance with the new configuration of energy, and the tensions and their related symptoms will be able to be released.

To see how this happens, we must look at further levels of detail of the consciousness, the energy system, and also the physical body.

One day, I was asked to visit a patient in a hospital who had fallen down an elevator shaft. Upon impact, her body was broken in several places, and her spinal cord was damaged. She was paralyzed and felt nothing below the chest, so when I touched her on different parts of her body, she felt nothing. When I moved my hand alongside her leg, without touching her leg, she described a sensation as if a wave were moving down her leg. There was no basis for any physical sensation, since I was not touching her. When I did touch her, she did not feel it because of the damage to her spinal cord.

To have a coherent explanation of how she could experience what she did, we can imagine her as an energy body occupying a physical body, and further imagine that the energy body had become separated from the physical body, so that she could experience and feel the energy body, but not the physical body.

Everything that we experience, we experience through the energy body. When the energy body and the physical body occupy the same space, there are parallel processes on the physical level, such as nerves being stimulated, electro-chemical reactions, electrical impulses moving along the nerves, etc. The physical sciences study the processes on the physical level, but these are not necessary to the experience at the level of consciousness. When someone experiences their consciousness in another place, as in dreams or astral travel, the other place is experienced as if with the physical senses, but the organs of the physical senses are not involved. The memories of the experience, however, can be stored on the physical level.

The physical sciences are based on the idea that the causes of symptoms are outside us (germs cause disease, accidents cause injuries, etc.). However, according to metaphysical principles, these things only happen when the proper conditions for them to happen exist in the consciousness. Metaphysically, we say that everything that happens on the physical level is an effect, and that the cause exists in the consciousness.

The physical model does not contradict the metaphysical, but rather describes the parallel processes that happen on the physical level when the conditions of consciousness have created the proper environment.

The consciousness does not occupy only the brain, but rather the entire body, so that through your consciousness, you are in contact with every part of your body. In fact, your consciousness extends beyond your body, usually to a distance of one to two meters (four to six feet) in every direction (and some say, infinitely). This aspect of your consciousness, and therefore, your energy field, is known as your *aura*.

The outer portions of the aura, the energy field, are quite subtle, and the energy becomes more and more dense as we approach what we know as the physical body. We can see the aura as composed of different densities of energy, corresponding to the different levels of energy radiating from the different bodies (physical, emotional, mental, astral, etheric, buddhic, and causal) that interpenetrate each other, occupying the same space at different rates of vibration. These various bodies will be discussed in more detail in Chapter Twelve.

Since the density of energy increases as we approach what we call the physical body, we can choose to see the physical body as just the next denser form of energy.

With our orientation toward the physical, we have come to look at ourselves as each a biological structure, but if we look closely at the building blocks of matter, we are also able to see ourselves as structures of energy.

The smallest biological unit, the cell, is composed of molecules, which are composed of atoms (or ions). These are composed of particles (neutrons, protons, electrons) that are composed of smaller particles (quarks, neutrinos, gluons, etc.), which are in turn composed of tiny black holes and white holes, each with a positive charge or a negative charge.

Patterns of these black holes and white holes, energy, form the smallest of what we call particles in the physical universe. Patterns of these patterns form larger particles, and patterns of these form atoms. Patterns of atoms form molecules, and patterns of molecules form cells. Patterns of cells form tissue, and patterns of tissue form organs.

Patterns of organs form the organism. We can say, therefore, that the entire organism is composed of nothing but tiny black holes and white holes in a particular configuration. It's only energy.

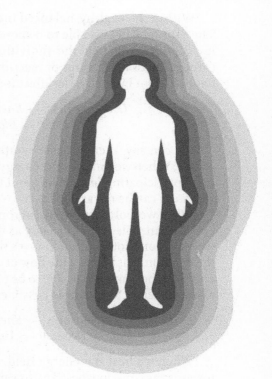

The Human Energy Field

From space, we see the earth moving around the sun, much as an electron moves around a nucleus. We can see the solar system as an atom, with about the same proportions of space to substance as an atom, existing in a larger molecule we call a galaxy. We can see other galaxies, other molecules, as part of a larger structure. And so on.

We are also able to see in space black holes and white holes (quasars). We see the same thing "out there" as we see "in there," and from a particular point of view, we have agreed to call what we see, "physical." It is just as easy to see it as only energy, and there is a benefit in doing that. When we do, we are not limited by the physical "laws." The words we use to describe our experience create our reality, so we are able to create healings, effects that seem to defy the physical "laws," because energy behaves differently from physical structure. It obeys different "laws."

When we see the physical structure as just a form of energy denser than the auras surrounding it, we can see ourselves as an energy system, composed of different densities of energy.

Within the healthy, balanced individual, the energy flows smoothly. The consciousness is able to respond successfully to each condition that it encounters. When the individual blocks the flow of this energy through certain decisions or reactions to conditions, and if the blockage has sufficient intensity, the effect is some symptom on the physical level.

Consciousness —> Energy Field —> Physical Body
Decision —> Blockage —> Symptom

We can say, then, that all symptoms are just reflections of blocked energy. When we unblock the energy through making a different decision or by participating in a healing and thus rebalancing the energy field, the symptom can be released.

When we look at our model of consciousness, energy field, and physical body, we are able to see the body as the end result of a process that begins with our consciousness and moves through our energy field. If we reverse the decision that blocked the flow of energy, the energy field returns to balance and the symptom is able to be released, according to whatever we can allow ourselves to believe is possible.

Consciousness —> Energy Field —> Physical Body
Change Decision —> Unblock —> Release Symptom

When we heal the energy field, the effects move in both directions, towards the consciousness and towards the physical, so that we experience a change in our consciousness (the stress on that level is released), and a release of tensions and symptoms on the physical level as well. The little black holes and the little white holes rearrange themselves. The biological structure rearranges itself, and the symptom is released. This happens either rapidly or slowly, again according to whatever we allow ourselves to believe is possible.

Consciousness <— Energy Field —> Physical Body
Tension Release <— Healing (Unblocking) —> Symptom Release

The symptom only served to communicate a condition to us. When the condition in consciousness no longer exists, the symptom has no further reason for being there.

Tension in a particular part of your body reflects tension in a particular part of your consciousness about a certain aspect of your life. The parts of your body that do not work well reflect the parts of your life that do not work well. When the tension about that part of your life can be released from that part of your consciousness, it can then be released from that part of your body. Your body, your consciousness, and that part of your life, are then able to return to their natural state of harmony. You return to the way of being that works best for you.

All illness, all injury is the result of blocked energy. Since we direct consciousness, or energy, with our thoughts, we have the ability to unblock the energy wherever it has been blocked in ourselves, or in others. When we do that, the result is a return to the experience of wholeness. Healing happens.

Obviously, then, anything can be healed.

CHAPTER 4

The Language of the Body

Somewhere within you, you have available to you a state of consciousness in which you are in perfect balance on all levels, experiencing perfect health. This is, in fact, your natural state of being.

When you experience this state of consciousness, you are responding to conditions in your life with optimal effectiveness, and you are in touch with your inner voice, your intuition, and are listening to it. You are being yourself. And you are healthy.

Your intuition speaks a very simple language: either it feels good, or it feels not-good. Everyone seems to agree that when you listen to your intuition, it always guides you to success. Therefore, you are being told to always do what feels good inside, and not do what feels not-good inside.

If you accept the idea that you have a purpose in life, you must also consider that it must be something that feels right for you to do. Otherwise, you would not be motivated to do it.

You are here to be happy. Therefore, you must do what makes you happy, and not do what makes you unhappy. If this is the rule at your deepest level of being, it must be true on all levels. Therefore, you are being told that you must do what you really want to do, and what feels good for you to do, and not do what you really don't want to do, what you feel resistance to doing. You are told to listen to your conscience.

When you do not listen to your inner voice, you experience unhappiness and tension. If you move more and more in the direction that feels not-good, you feel more and more resistance in your emotions, and in the tendency for events to not happen the way you want. When the resistance becomes strong enough, you may say to yourself, "I should have listened to that inner voice when it told me to do something different." Therefore, you must have heard the inner voice. Otherwise, you would not have been able to say, "I should have listened."

When you do what you know you should have done in the first place, there is a release of tension, you feel better, and you return to a state of harmony with yourself, as well as with your environment. If instead you continue to move in the direction that feels not-good, you experience more and more tension, more and more resistance, until the tension reaches the physical level, and you develop a physical symptom or attract experiences to yourself that result in a physical symptom. The symptom might then be the result of a disease, an "accident," a fall, a pinched nerve, etc.

For our purposes, the important thing to look at is the symptom, the effect. Metaphysically, we say that the end result that happened was the real original intention. The experience happened in order to have the end result.

There are no accidents, and no coincidences. If everything begins in your consciousness, then all that happens on the physical level is the result of what has been happening in your consciousness. If the effect of the event was a symptom, the event happened in order to create the symptom, because it was important for you to receive a message from your higher self that you had not been listening to at the level of intuition or emotion.

Symptoms speak to you in your own language, telling you what you have been doing to yourself. This language reflects the idea that you create your reality, totally. When you describe the symptom within this context, the metaphoric significance of the symptom becomes obvious.

Your body is then saying that this is what you have been doing to yourself, with the way of being you have chosen until now, with what you have been doing in your consciousness. The implication is that you may continue to maintain the same way of being, or do something different. It's not a question of right or wrong, but rather simple cause-and-effect. The process is not one involving guilt, but rather just acknowledging responsibility. One way of being creates a symptom. Another way of being releases the symptom. It is you who decide your way of being.

When you understand the message that your body has given you, and make the necessary changes in your consciousness and in your way of being, so that you are no longer doing what has been out of balance, what is not right for you, then you return to harmony on all levels.

The symptom, which served only to give a message, has no further reason for existing, and so it can be released, in accordance with your sensitivities and belief systems, and therefore with what you can allow yourself to believe is possible.

All of this must be examined within the context of what was happening in your life at the time that the symptom developed, since it was your response to these conditions that created the symptom.

Within my own experience, I had had cancer of the spinal cord, at the level of the neck. I was terminally ill. My symptoms were paralysis, inability to walk, and a lot of pain.

Cancer represents something held in, and not expressed. When we hold something in without expressing it, it grows and grows inside us.

This is a perfect metaphor for cancer. The part of the body affected shows what has been held in and not expressed.

For me, the cancer had been in the part of my energy system representing communication and expression. I had been keeping myself from expressing what was true for me. I had been in an unhappy marriage in which I had not felt free to communicate without it becoming an argument.

When I describe my symptoms from the point of view that I created them, then rather than saying that I was paralyzed, I would have to say that I had been paralyzing myself. I had been trying to be what I thought others wanted me to be, rather than being myself. The real me was inside, but I had not been letting the real me express my true being. By doing that, I had been causing myself much pain.

Rather than saying that I couldn't walk, I had to say that I had been keeping myself from walking. I had been keeping myself in experiences in which I was unhappy, and keeping myself from walking away, when that was what I had really wanted to do. The effects of the stress I experienced because of that had reached catastrophic proportions in my body.

I realized that in order to release the symptoms, I had to release the way of being that had created the symptoms. Rather than saying that I was dying, I had to say that I had been killing myself. I had to acknowledge that, according to the idea that everything begins with a decision in our consciousness, any terminal illness must begin with a decision to die. Therefore, I had decided to die. People die for one of two reasons. Either their trip is over, and they have experienced or accomplished what they wanted to in their lifetime and are therefore complete, or they are in a situation or experience that is difficult, and they see no way out of the situation, other than to die. The latter was true for me.

I realized that for me to continue to live, I would have to express the real me, communicate what is true for me, leave the situations in which I had been unhappy, and consider alternatives to the lifestyle in which I had been killing myself. I would also have to consider alternatives to the standard medical model in which my situation was considered hopeless. I did all of that, and changed my life.

Since the medical model presented no solution, I received no treatment, and no medication. Since I was expected to die any minute if I coughed or sneezed, each meal was the last one I might ever experience, and so I ate whatever I wanted, and loved it. I had no special diet. What I happened to desire at that time, and enjoy, was a lot of hamburgers, sausages, pizza, and Coca-Cola. Therefore, what I needed at that time was a lot of yang energy and a wide yin-yang spectrum.

What I changed was my mental diet, the ideas I chose to accept into my consciousness. When I had a certain thought and felt bad afterward, I knew that I was creating stress by choosing that thought. Stress creates illness. If I wanted to feel better, I knew that I had to choose different thoughts that felt better.

I took responsibility for my condition. I acknowledged to myself the importance of being happy, and of doing what makes me happy. I also dedicated myself to the inner work that was necessary to allow myself to believe that the symptom was being released. The effects were that the hopeless condition was reversed. The healing happened.

The process took me two months of intensive work on myself, because I believed that it would take two months. I didn't know then what I know now. With the tools presented with the Body Mirror System, the same thing can be accomplished in two weeks, or even two hours. In fact, the moment of change from a state of deterioration to a state of improvement takes only an instant. After that, one only needs to hold the perception that the healing is underway, and happening, and notice the improvements on the physical level as they present themselves.

The important thing is to realize that anything can be healed. It isn't a question of whether or not it can happen, but rather just one of knowing how to do it.

Then, just do it.

When you understand the language of your body, you will be able to listen to the messages earlier and earlier, until you are functioning fully in accord with your inner being, your higher self. At that time, it will be possible to no longer concern yourself with healing, because there will be no further need for you to receive the messages through symptoms. You will be able to function more and more from your center, listening to your inner voice, and doing what is right for you to do.

You will be healthier. And a lot happier.

Anything can be healed.

The Body Mirror System

Concepts and Tools

CHAPTER 5

The Chakras

Chakra is a Sanskrit word meaning "wheel," or vortex, and it refers to each of the seven energy centers of which your consciousness, your energy system, is composed.

Your consciousness represents all that it is possible for you to experience. All your perceptions, all your senses, all your thought processes, and all states of being of which you are capable, happen within what is called your consciousness. Your consciousness can be divided into seven categories, and each of these is associated with a particular energy center, or chakra.

Your consciousness is an energy system. It is composed of different densities of energy in a state of flow, of movement. When the energy flows smoothly, you experience wholeness. When the energy is blocked, you experience tension, which can manifest as symptoms. The chakras function as pumps, or valves, regulating the flow of energy through your energy system. The state of flow of the energy of your consciousness is therefore determined by the state of your chakras.

The functioning of the chakras reflects decisions you make concerning how you choose to respond to conditions in your life. You open and close these valves when you decide what to think, and what to feel, and through which perceptual filter you choose to experience the world around you. The idea, of course, is to keep all of the valves working smoothly, like the valves of a flute. When there is residual tension in your consciousness about something that has happened in your life, it is as though this tension affects the smooth functioning of the valves in your energy system. They can get "stuck," and therefore not open and close so smoothly.

The chakras are aspects of consciousness, as are the auras. The chakras are more dense than the auras, but not as dense as the physical body. They are like solid balls of energy interpenetrating the physical body, as a magnetic field can interpenetrate the physical body.

Each of the chakras is associated with one of the endocrine glands, and also with a certain group of nerves, a *plexus*. When you experience tension in a certain part of your consciousness, you experience it in the chakra associated with that part of your consciousness. The tension is then

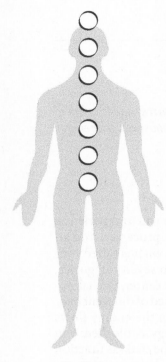

The Chakras

transmitted to the endocrine gland associated with that chakra. The endocrine glands secrete hormones, which change the chemistry of the body. Thus, a change in consciousness creates a change in body chemistry, depending upon the needs of the moment.

For example, if you are walking through a forest and you meet a bear, the perception of a threat to survival will stimulate the secretion of adrenalin, preparing your body to fight or run. Perceptions concerning survival are associated with the Red Chakra, also called the Root Chakra, and the adrenal glands are also associated with this chakra. Thus, we can say that the tension of the perceived threat to survival was experienced in the Red Chakra, which transmitted the tension to the adrenal glands, which responded to the perceived threat by secreting adrenalin.

The tension is also transmitted, via the chakra concerned, to the nerve plexus associated with that chakra, and thus to the parts of the body controlled by that plexus, that group of nerves. The Red Chakra controls the legs, through the sacral plexus. With the example given (meeting a bear), we can say that the tension concerning the perceived threat to survival was transmitted by the Red Chakra through the sacral plexus to the legs, which were then energized for running. Tensions in the body can thus be associated with specific tensions in the consciousness. In this way, the body can be seen as a map of the consciousness within.

As an exercise you can do now, imagine a situation about which you feel or have felt some tension. As you think of the situation and feel whatever you feel about it, notice where in your body you feel the tension. If you were to draw a circle around that part of the body, how large would the circle be?

If you were to imagine a particular color within the circle, what color would you imagine?

If you were to describe the physical sensations you experience within the circle, what words would you use? (You can describe the tension as resistance to the flow of energy, a place where you have been resisting the flow of energy through your energy system.)

If you have been resisting the flow of energy, you can also remove the resistance, consciously relaxing the place you have been holding tense. As you do this more and more, you can feel that part of your body relaxing again, opening more and more to the flow of energy, until you again experience yourself being clear and comfortable, a clear channel for the flow of energy once more.

Where you felt the tension depended on why you felt the tension. Thus, if the resistance was experienced at the level of the perineum, between your anus and your sex organs, it was because of tension in your consciousness concerned with security, survival, and trust. For most people, this represents their relationship with money, home, and job. If the resistance was felt at the level of the abdomen, the tension had something to do with perceptions concerning food or sex. If it was felt at the level of the solar plexus, it had to do with perceptions concerning power, control, and your freedom to be yourself.

If it was felt at the level of the heart, the tension had something to do with your perceptions of love, and the area of relationships in your life. If it was felt at the level of the throat, the tension was there because of something that you wanted to express but didn't.

If you felt the tension in your forehead, it was because of feeling that you were not being seen for who you are, but rather the role you were in, and if you felt the tension at the top of your head, it was because of feeling separate when you wanted to feel connected, or feeling connected when you wanted to feel separate, or a problem with authority.

If such statements accurately describe what you experienced, then we can say that the tensions you felt in your consciousness were being experienced in the energy centers that represent your consciousness—your chakras. You have always been able to feel your chakras. You just have not been taught to examine your experiences in this way.

The chakras have been studied for thousands of years, often for their esoteric significance, and for the special states of consciousness they represent, states of consciousness considered non-ordinary. We see here, though, that they also have a very practical, everyday use; they show us through our body what we have been experiencing in our consciousness.

When the tension in your consciousness (and, therefore, in your chakras) reaches a particular level of intensity, or continues for a period of time, the tension is communicated through the nerve groups to the parts of the body controlled by those nerve groups. Consequently those parts of the body and functions in the body controlled by those nerve groups can be affected. You can then develop symptoms that reflect what you have been doing to yourself, when you describe the symptoms in a way that reflects the idea that you have created them.

Each chakra is associated with a particular element, a particular sense, and specific systems within the body. It is only when tensions in the consciousness reach a certain intensity that they result in physical symptoms. Symptoms can therefore be read, to understand what parts of the consciousness have been experiencing tension, and need to change in order for the individual to return to a state of wholeness. (See Appendix 1—The Chakra Healing Guide.)

It must be remembered that the chakras are only parts of your consciousness, and that it is you who decide the state of your chakras. As you dance through the conditions that present themselves to you in your life, you decide how to respond. You therefore open and close your chakras, playing these valves as a musician would play the valves in a flute. It is obviously important that none of the valves is stuck open or stuck closed, since that would leave you stuck at the effect of previous patterns of responding.

It is only when all chakras function freely as they should, that you are able to examine each situation in your life consciously, deciding in that moment the proper course of action, and the response you choose to make. Then, you are really free.

The implication is that you have within you, and available to you, a state of consciousness in which you experience your wholeness, and you function optimally. It is a state we can call perfection.

When you experience this state, you can continue to function until your job is done and you choose to leave the planet. However, until that time, the question is one of how you choose to experience yourself, in comfort (ease) or dis-ease, and also how long you choose to wait until you go for perfection and optimal functioning.

If you have been experiencing symptoms until now, you can resolve to do what is necessary to return to balance, reminding yourself that anything can be healed, and that it is you who decide what happens in your consciousness, and therefore, in your body.

Many of those on the spiritual path seek enlightenment, but it should be remembered that enlightenment is not perfection. There are enlightened beings who still experience symptoms, which means that they are not experiencing all of their consciousness, all of their energy system, with clarity. There are also beings who are functioning perfectly, but who may not have experienced the state known as enlightenment. It merely means that whatever these beings have been doing instinctively has been working for them.

While the chakras are often associated with various spiritual practices and processes of accelerated evolution, it should be mentioned that here the chakras are explored simply as a map of consciousness, and as tools, which can be used within a technology of healing. The intention is always to return to balance when necessary, and to understand enough about how our consciousness works, so that we have a tendency to remain in balance, and to accept this as our natural state.

Some say that the key to happiness is a path of nonattachment, avoiding attachments or aversions that keep you from fully experiencing the present moment of life, and what it offers.

An attachment is about needing to have something, whereas an aversion, or negative attachment, is about needing to not have something. Both are attachments, and either can manifest in your consciousness as being occupied with something, needing to have it or needing to avoid it, to the point where the tension in the consciousness is experienced as a constant preoccupation, like an addiction. In that way, attachment, being always present as a tension in the background, can be an interference to experiencing the present moment, the here and now of where you are.

When you are attached to something and you don't have it, you feel bad, and the degree of resistance that you feel shows how much you were attached, or addicted. The attachment can be at the level of any chakra, and a constant tension in a chakra can be seen as either a need to release this tension at the level of that chakra by resolving something in your life, or as a need to release an attachment to something in order to be able to enjoy the here and now of life.

Later chapters in this book will describe methods of releasing these attachments or aversions. We are always working relative to where you are, in your development. If you are in the first grade of school, the only question that concerns us is whether you are equipped to function at that level. If you are a postgraduate university student, we are still only concerned with whether you can function optimally at that level of the perpetual learning experience we call Life.

If something works well, leave it alone.

If it doesn't work, heal it.

Anything can be healed.

CHAPTER 6

Other Aspects of the Chakras

Each of the chakras is energy vibrating at a certain frequency, in relationship with other chakras vibrating at other frequencies, in a logical, orderly sequence of seven vibrations.

Within this sequence of seven vibrations, the heaviest, the most dense, is at the bottom, and the lightest is on top. Each chakra is associated with a certain element, and the sequence of these elements follows the same logic and order. The heaviest element, earth, is associated with the Root or Red Chakra, at the bottom. Water, which is lighter than earth, is associated with the second chakra, the Orange Chakra. These are followed in turn by the elements of fire, air, ether, inner sound, and inner light associated with the remaining chakras, in order of increasing lightness.

By observing your relationship with the different elements, you are able to see your relationship with the parts of your consciousness associated with those elements. For example, someone who does not have a clear relationship with water, may be afraid to swim or to be on a boat, and the way they feel about water can be seen to reflect their feelings about the parts of their consciousness that water represents (food and sex).

Each of the chakras is also associated with a certain level of experience. From the point of view that you are a consciousness in a body, your deepest inner experience is at the level we call the soul, and your outermost level of experience is at the boundaries of your physical body. Each of the levels of experience between these two is associated with a different subtle body, and each subtle body is associated with a particular chakra.

Thus, the Red Chakra is associated with the most dense body, the physical. The Orange Chakra is associated with the emotional body, which is the next lightest. These are followed by the Yellow Chakra, at the level of the solar plexus, associated with the mental body; the Green or Heart Chakra with the astral body; the Blue or Throat Chakra with the etheric body; the Brow or Indigo Chakra with the Buddhic (the Spirit); and the Crown or Violet Chakra with the causal body (the soul).

You can see that each level of being, and therefore each subtle body, is associated with a particular chakra. The evolution of your soul can be seen as learning to live from deeper and deeper parts of your being, until you live from your soul, rather than from the level that society considers normal, which is far from the deepest part of your being. Those who have learned to do this, and who live from these deepest levels, are considered extraordinary beings, whom we call evolved.

Since the chakras are each associated with a particular level of being, the evolution of your soul can be said to be represented by the chakras, which also show you everything that is happening in your consciousness.

If the evolution of your soul and the understanding of the nature of your consciousness are your main reasons for being on earth, the goals of your movie in which you are the main character, then everything in the movie must be about that. You can look around yourself and ask yourself what you are being shown about your inner being and the evolution of your soul, and about what is happening in your consciousness.

You can see other examples of energy vibrating at different frequencies in a logical, orderly sequence of seven, and you can consider the possibility that these other examples of seven vibrations must tell you something about yourself. You can see, for example, that the rainbow is a series of seven vibrations—colors—in a logical and orderly sequence. If the longest wavelength, the heaviest color, red, is associated with the lowest chakra (Root Chakra), and the shortest wavelength, the lightest color, violet, with the highest chakra (Crown Chakra), each of the colors can be used to represent a chakra in its clear state.

You can then see that your relationship with a particular color reflects your relationship with the part of your consciousness that the color represents. The colors of the spectrum, then, represent the different parts of human consciousness, as well as being a universal language that is deep within each person's consciousness.

Many people do not know that they know this language, but since the way they speak of their relationships with the colors accurately describes their relationship with the corresponding parts of their consciousness, we can see that somewhere inside, they must know this language well.

We can refer to the chakras, then, by their associated colors—Red, Orange, Yellow, Green, Blue, Indigo, and Violet.

In addition to the vertical scale that the chakras represent, from the perineum to the top of the head, we can also look at ourselves in terms of the polarity of yang and yin, or our male and female characteristics.

For most people, their right side is their yang side, and represents characteristics considered masculine. Their left side is their yin side, and represents characteristics considered feminine. For people who were born left-handed, this polarity is reversed, and their left side is their yang side, while their right side is their yin side.

The polarity, then, can be described as yang and yin, male and female, will and spirit, acting and feeling, intellect and emotions, etc. If parts of the body are described in this way, we can then refer to the will leg and the feeling leg, or the male leg and the female leg, and so on.

In Appendix 1, The Chakra Healing Guide, various aspects of the chakras are described in detail, within the context of healing, and symptoms associated with an imbalance or tension in each chakra are given. By studying the Guide you can gain a deeper understanding of the chakras, what they represent and how they are involved with our state of balance and health.

Thus a map of consciousness can be created. Tensions in the chakras can be released, and symptoms can be healed.

Anything can be healed.

CHAPTER 7

The White Light

When you are in the deepest part of your being, as a single point of consciousness glowing with intelligence, you experience the White Light. In other words, the deepest part of who you are is the source of the White Light, although some people choose to experience it as coming from above.

It is because it comes from and represents this deepest part of yourself that it can be used for cleansing and releasing all that is not you. Some healers like to cleanse themselves after a healing, if they feel they have taken on the subject's vibration or consciousness. If this is true for you, you can do this by filling yourself with your own White Light, and returning to the consciousness you know and recognize as yourself when you are in balance.

White Light is known esoterically as the highest form of spiritual protection, and it often is used to create the perception of being protected from perceived threats. When you fill yourself with White Light, and surround yourself with White Light, you can feel protected. When you experience this, you feel safe and more relaxed. When you relax more, and open more, you glow with more White Light, and feel safer. This process continues until you are totally open, and totally relaxed, and feeling totally protected, and totally in the White Light.

When you have a perception of someone else as having a problem, or a potential problem ("I'm worried about so-and-so and I hope they are okay."), you can imagine the person filled with White Light and surrounded by White Light, and hold the perception that the person is, in fact, all right. Your perceptions create your reality. Rather than continuing to hold the perception of the problem, you can see the other in the White Light, happy and healthy, and doing something they love to do. By insisting on holding that perception, you thereby contribute that image to the co-creation we call physical external reality.

Since we are each a consciousness, with the same spiritual equipment and abilities, we are all equal beings spiritually. No one has power over you, unless you have given them that power with your perceptions. When you fear another, the perception of fear, of feeling threatened, is what gives the power to the other. The resistance, the fear, is the mechanism for that. If you did not fear the other, you would not be holding the perception that they were more powerful than you. If you did not perceive them as more powerful than you, there would be nothing to fear.

When you put yourself in the White Light, and put the other in the White Light as well, a perception of equality is created, as well as a basis for communication without the perception of feeling threatened. The resistance has been removed, and clarity in the consciousness can be experienced. It is in this way that some healers prefer to communicate with spirits, without feeling threatened by those spirits. To do this, you can fill and surround yourself with White Light, and see the spirit filled and surrounded with White Light, and then you are able to ask, "Who are you, and what do you want?" After all, there must be a positive reason why a spirit has chosen to present itself for communication. Sometimes, it just wants you to know that it's there, and watching, as might be the case with a relative who has crossed over, like a father whose spirit wants his child to know that she is not alone, even though her father has "died."

Sometimes, spirits are there to help, or to give information, or a view from the other side, which can be helpful. And sometimes, they need help with resolving something that has been incomplete, so that they can continue their journey. Healing has many forms.

Since white light is made up of all of the colors of the spectrum, we can say that the consciousness, whose parts are composed of all of the chakras together, of all of the colors combined, can be referred to as White Light. White Light, then, represents the consciousness that is deciding which chakra to look through and experience at that time, or which channel it chooses to watch on its television set.

In 1975, during the unsuccessful operation that was intended to remove the tumor from my spinal cord, I went through the tunnel that people speak of when they describe the process of leaving the body at the time of death, or during what are known as "near death experiences."

I met a Being of Light on the other side who was there to let me know that it was time for me to move on. The Being had no human form, but was rather just a spark of consciousness glowing with energy and intelligence, and I experienced myself as that, too. Within the philosophical spiritual structure in which I believe, we are each that, in the deepest part of our being, at the level we call the soul. We are each light, White Light manifesting.

Sometimes, if we close the Violet Chakra through not perceiving ourselves as loved by our father, we may give ourselves reasons for that perception ("I'm not worthy of love," or "I'm no good," or "I did something wrong and now I have to be punished," etc.), and then we live at the effect of those decisions. Since the Violet Chakra represents the deepest part of who we are, as light, we can say that we are keeping ourselves from perceiving ourselves as that light.

We may build a personification based on the misperception, an image of ourselves as shadow beings, or beings of darkness. Then, the difficulty in our relationship with our father is reflected in our difficulties that we have experiencing the White Light, for example in meditation, until we can again open to it. Then we can experience what we consider redemption, once more allowing in the love of our father.

Since White Light represents the deepest part of who we each are, it represents that part of us that exists behind and beyond any symptoms. The symptoms are not who we are, but just what we have been experiencing, and not from our deepest part.

When healers see their subject filled with White Light, they are then able to insist on holding their perceptions on that deepest level of the subject. It should be remembered that the healing is being created in the perceptions of the healer, and is then agreed to by the subject. Here, the White Light is being used as a trigger mechanism to create the perception that the other is healed.

Similarly, if you are feeling yourself caught in some movie, experiencing yourself at the effect of some symptoms, or of some experiences other than your wholeness, you can remind yourself of who you are, really, by dropping into your center and experiencing yourself as the Being of Light that you are. As you do this, you can identify more and more with this level of being, until it is a new habit, and your new usual way of being.

You choose whatever perceptions may be necessary in order to watch the release of the symptoms, and identify more and more with the experience of your wholeness. You are able to identify more and more with the God within, the light within, the source within, being That which you are.

To say, "I Am," you must just be.

Just be.

And know that anything can be healed.

CHAPTER 8

Passage

Each of the chakras is like a lens through which you choose to interpret events in the outer world. You always have the choice as to whether you will interpret these events through the filter of security, sensation, freedom or power, love, expression or abundance, spirit, or unity.

When you look through a particular filter, or chakra, it's as though you're in the center of a bubble colored by that filter, and all information coming into your consciousness must pass through that bubble. It can then seem as though your perceptions are reflections of what is universally true, and that everyone you see has their motivations in that same chakra.

When your primary consideration in a particular moment is security, for example, we can say that you are looking at the world through the Red Chakra. It then seems as though everyone is motivated by security, or feeling threatened by its lack. You are not necessarily seeing the world the way it is, but rather as *you* are.

As your motivations change, so does your filter. When your motivation is sensation, for example, events in the outer world make sense in another way than they did through the filter of security. You may have noticed that sometimes, when your desire for sensation has been satisfied, you have been surprised at how differently you saw things the next morning.

All day long, you are moving through your chakras, seeing through different filters, depending on what you choose as your motivation in any moment. You always have seven programs playing on your television set, seven different apparent scenarios, and you are always choosing which program to watch at any time. The idea is to not have static or interference on any of the channels. When you are seeing through a chakra in which you have tensions, the picture is distorted by those tensions. When the tensions are removed, so is the distortion. As with any television set, if you do not like the program you are watching, you can just switch channels, by deciding to look through a different chakra to see a different scenario.

We can say that one of the chakras is your *home*. You decide what your home is when you choose your primary motivating force during that period of your life. You can see, for that period, the thing that is most important to you, your main reason for doing things, and you will know which chakra is your home.

From your home, you travel through the other chakras, depending on your motivations in any particular moment, and then you return to your "background" state of consciousness, your home. It is the place where your consciousness stays when there is nothing happening for you in a particular moment that takes your attention to another place.

When you change the primary motivating force in your life, you move your home state of consciousness. This always involves a corresponding shift in your perceptions. The move from the Yellow Chakra (the Solar Plexus Chakra, or Power Center) to the Green Chakra (the Heart Chakra, or Living Love Center) involves a particularly large shift. For many people, it is as though there is a membrane between those two chakras, and on the physical level, it corresponds to the diaphragm.

Below the membrane are the three lower chakras, and the perceptions at these levels are considered ordinary by society's standards. Our society has defined normal perceptions as those motivated by security, sensation, and power. Perceptions through the higher chakras are considered non-ordinary perceptions, and are often seen as unusual or mystical states of consciousness.

We have mentioned before that the chakras represent a logical and orderly sequence of seven vibrations, and that, therefore, other orderly sequences of seven vibrations in the world around us can be seen as representing the evolution of our soul, telling us something about our consciousness. The seven notes of the musical scale (Do, Re, Mi, Fa, Sol, La, Ti) are a sequence of seven vibrations in a logical order, and each note can be associated with a particular chakra. Music played in a particular key vibrates a particular chakra, and evokes a particular emotion.

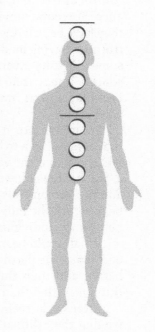

There is a precise mathematical relationship that exists between the frequencies that each note represents. It is a mathematical progression. Within that mathematical progression, however, there are two places where it does something different. The smooth progression is interrupted. In Nada Yoga, for example, each note is divided into several parts, as follows: Do = 4 beats, Re = 3 beats, Mi = 2 beats, Fa = 4 beats, Sol = 4 beats, La = 3 beats, Ti = 2 beats, Do = 4 beats, etc. Thus, 4 - 3 - 2 - 4 - 4 - 3 - 2 - 4, etc.

Evolutionary Shock Points

There is a shift in register between Mi and Fa, and between Ti and the first Do of the next octave.

We can say, then, that the shift occurs between the Yellow Chakra and the Green Chakra, and also above the Violet Chakra. According to the philosopher Gurdjieff, when the chakras are seen as representing human evolution, these two shift regions are considered shock points, membranes that we must pass through in our process of evolution. The process may be rough or gentle, depending on the perceptions we choose.

For the passage through the membrane between the Yellow Chakra and the Green Chakra, perceptual changes are necessary to open clearer perceptions of love. For the passage through the Violet Chakra membrane, the perceptions must be aligned to resolve the apparent paradox or conflict between concepts of autonomy and accord with authority.

When someone decides to move through either of these membranes, it takes some time for all of their perceptions to be aligned with their decision to evolve. During that time, they recognize more and more the new priorities that are the bases for their decisions. They are also still responding to the conditions in their life that have been stimulated by their deep inner decision.

Perceptions at the level of the Yellow Chakra may be concerned with control or freedom, and those of the Green Chakra with love and acceptance. Someone moving from the Yellow Chakra to the Green Chakra, if they have been living the aspect of control, and are still holding on to control after having made the decision to evolve to acceptance, may experience some difficulty. Events in their life will seem to go more and more out of control. It may seem as though the world is coming to an end, and destruction may appear imminent, until they let go of control, and open up to acceptance.

Sometimes, to stimulate the opening to acceptance, there is a shock that obliges them to let go. The shock may be physical or emotional. When it is emotional and very strong, it may be experienced as what is known as a "mental breakdown," where the mental cognitive processes break down and the person feels out of control. While the traditional treatment may be to return the individual to their "normal" perceptions, this may not be best for the individual in their process of evolution.

What would be much better, and quicker as well as easier, would be to encourage the person to put their attention on new perceptions that feel better, and then this spiritual process will be experienced as a breakthrough, rather than a breakdown.

Afterwards, seeing life from the new point of view, the person can realize that their difficulties were the result of the degree to which they had held on to control. They will see that in that way, they had created their own discomfort, and their own pain. They will be able to see themselves (as they had been) with compassion, and they will no longer feel the need to defend a way of being that did not work for them, and that, in fact, no longer exists.

During extreme examples of a difficult passage, the individual may feel as though they are dying. Although the feeling is real, there is no danger here of mortality. It is simply a process going on in the consciousness. The person had identified themselves with a particular way of being, while at the same time desiring to see things in a different way. For things to make sense in a new way, of course, they must no longer make sense in the old way. It is the old way of being which is dying.

If the person persists in holding to the old view, and the old personification, they may experience the process that happens as an "ego death." This will be true as long as they maintain the perspective toward the past and what is being let go of. If the focus is shifted to the present, with an orientation toward the future, the person becomes aware of the new way of being that is emerging, and the same process is experienced as a rebirth.

We can look at the process as one of moving from one reality to another, or from one bubble to another. If we imagine these as soap bubbles that are touching, we can see the membrane that exists where the two bubbles meet, as representing the membrane we have been talking about.

From the old bubble, there were certain perceptions with which the person has identified themselves. They could say, "This is me. I define myself

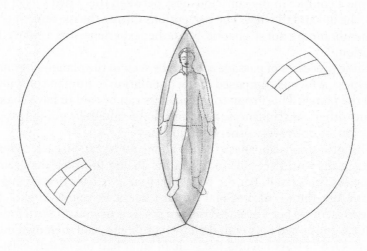

Moving through the Membrane

with these perceptions, but I want things to make sense in another way." With this desire to change, they begin the movement out of one bubble, toward the other. They reach the membrane between the two, where things no longer make sense in the old way, and do not yet make sense in the new way. During that narrow slice of time, during the passage through the energy field represented as the membrane between the two bubbles, their perceptions may be those of chaos and confusion, until the entry into the new bubble has begun.

If the individual orients their perceptions toward the past, to the way things used to make sense, it doesn't work. The person doing this becomes aware of the things they must let go of. The idea, then, is to recognize the process as one of passage, and orient the perceptions toward the future, the new bubble.

As that happens, new perceptions present themselves, and emerge from the new reality. Things begin to make sense, but in a way different than before. As movement into the new bubble continues, the process continues, and the individual is able to define themselves in terms of their new perceptions, experiencing the process as a rebirth. Someone going through this process with difficulty may feel a sense of physical pressure between the solar plexus and the heart, at the level of the membrane, and it can be extreme, but at the same time, easy to release during a healing.

The process is much gentler when the person has been living the aspect of freedom, rather than control, in the solar plexus chakra. The transition from freedom to acceptance is a lot easier than the transition from control to acceptance. In moving from freedom to acceptance, there is not so extreme a conflict in the consciousness between these two sets of perceptions, the old and the new. The perceptions during the movement through the membrane are not so chaotic, but rather experienced as a gentle, logical evolution.

These processes of passage can also be seen in the planetary group consciousness, which is composed of the population of human consciousness upon the planet. This group consciousness can be said to have chakras, as can any other consciousness, and can also be said to be going through its evolution, as does every other consciousness.

This group consciousness spends about 2000 years in each chakra, and events in the world are able to reflect the chakra in which the group consciousness finds itself. For the past 2000 years, we have been living in the Piscean Age, the age of the Solar Plexus Chakra, or Yellow Chakra. Events in the world have been oriented toward power and control, with individual countries concerned only with their own problems, and their own interests. This has led to wars beyond the scale of what had previously existed. We have developed enough power to destroy ourselves, many times over.

When the Being known as Jesus walked the earth 2000 years ago, he represented the aspect of the Heart Chakra, or Green Chakra, which at the time was not at all common. What he saw as he looked around himself was evidence of Yellow Chakra disorders. (The Yellow Chakra controls the skin, among other things.) Leprosy was prevalent, a skin condition in which the face deteriorates. The symptoms, people hiding their faces, imply guilt as the underlying way of being creating the physical condition, and it is then easy to understand the desire on the part of the Being, Jesus, to free humanity from this self-imposed and unnecessary burden.

Now, we have entered what some call the Age of Aquarius, the age of the Heart Chakra, the Green Chakra, and conditions around us are obliging us to put our attention on Green Chakra perceptions. For example, we have created the disease of AIDS as a condition of our times. While the medical community continues to seek solutions on the physical level for this affliction, the alternative community has been having some success with healing this disease through changing the individual's perceptions of love.

Nations are now more concerned with global awareness and our role as a global community. We have become obliged to look beyond national boundaries, and the shocks of past and present outrages are motivating us to do something different from what we have done before.

There are still some who have not yet made this passage, and their perceptions have been presenting them with images of global catastrophes, but these can be seen as events designed to stimulate an increasing sense of global community, if it does not happen in a gentler manner.

These perceptions can also be seen as the natural effects of seeing through the filter of the Yellow Chakra, and of course, will give way to new perceptions of global awareness and the necessity of serving each others' needs in order for our own needs to be served, when seen from the more evolved view of the Green Chakra.

Because this is all happening on a global level, it is happening to more and more individuals within the group consciousness. More and more individuals are making the passage from the Yellow Chakra to the Green Chakra. The more beings that make this passage, the more effect it has, at an accelerating rate, on the rest of the group consciousness, until the movement is complete, and we are able to function effectively as a global community, the members of which have found a way to live together harmoniously. Then, the healing will have been complete.

At that time, perhaps, if there is indeed a larger community of beings, within which humanity and life on planet earth is only a small part, we can be approached by them without our feeling threatened, and perhaps we can then be considered ready for active membership with them in that community.

Anything can be healed.

CHAPTER 9

Thought Forms

When people are not experiencing their wellness, when they are experiencing a symptom, sometimes they describe the symptom as if it is a thing.

People may say that the symptom feels like a heavy weight sitting on their head, or like a sharp knife in their side. In terms of what they are experiencing, there is a thing there, and it feels as real to them, as if it existed in the physical universe.

We are working with the idea that these thoughts are things, and that they are, in fact, real. They exist as thought forms at the level we know as the ether, the crossover between the physical and spiritual universes. The ether, from the esoteric point of view, from the spiritual universe, is the matrix on which the physical universe is projected. Our thoughts, our goals, the pictures we create with our consciousness and put into our consciousness are said to go into the ether, as holographic images, waiting to manifest in the physical world when conditions are appropriate.

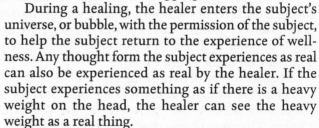

During a healing, the healer enters the subject's universe, or bubble, with the permission of the subject, to help the subject return to the experience of wellness. Any thought form the subject experiences as real can also be experienced as real by the healer. If the subject experiences something as if there is a heavy weight on the head, the healer can see the heavy weight as a real thing.

The thought form, at the etheric level, can be said to be made of energy. The healer is able to see the energy and feel it. The more senses that healers can focus on the thought form that is there, the more real they are able to make it to themselves. When the thought form is as real to the healer as it is to the subject who is experiencing the symptom, the healer can then remove the thought form from the experience of the subject. As the subject feels the thought form

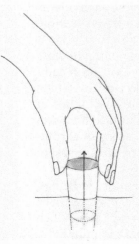

Removing the Hole

leave, they are again able to return to the experience of wholeness. If there was a biological basis for the symptom and the experience of the thought form, and the symptom and thought form have been released and are no longer being experienced, the biological basis must also have been released.

If a subject experiences a headache that feels like a heavy weight on the head, you as the healer can decide that you see and feel the weight, and when you experience it as a real thing, you are then able to remove it. When you do that, the experience that was called a headache is no longer felt. The subject feels it leave, and returns to the experience of wellness. If there was an organic basis for the headache, that organic basis must have been released at the same time.

If the subject reports an experience like a sharp knife, then there is a sharp knife. You can decide to feel it, and see it, and then remove it from the experience of the subject. In doing that, the healing happens.

You must, while working in this way, treat these things as real. For example, when the knife was removed, one can imagine that it left a hole, and then something must be done about the hole. You can fill the hole, seal the hole, sew up the hole, or even remove the hole. After all, the hole is a thing, too. If we start with a hole in a subject, and we remove the hole, we are left with a subject without the hole. They are whole.

There is no limit to what can be done while working in the etheric plane of existence. You can imagine any story you want to, and insist on allowing yourself to believe the story you know you are imagining. When you do that, the healing happens. Shamanic healers work in this way, seeing symptoms as stones, worms, or other objects that they remove from the body, creating in themselves the perception that the healing has happened. The psychic surgeons in the Philippines and in South America work in the very same way.

When these things are treated as real, something must be done with them when they are removed from the subject. Since the words you use to describe your experience create your reality, you can decide that this object, when thrown to the floor, will self-destruct in two seconds, and you can watch it do that. Or, you can decide to return this thing to the big ball of energy from which all things come, or you can decide that the sensations you experience while holding this thing can be re-interpreted in another way, for example, as intense White Light that will be useful for the healing.

Continuing with our earlier example, when you remove the hole from the subject, leaving the subject whole, you can save the hole and put it in your pocket. If you later find yourself working with someone with an enormous stone wall around the heart, for example, you can remove the hole from your pocket and put it into the wall. Then, there is a hole in the wall that you can use to make contact. A hole can be a useful tool. Obviously,

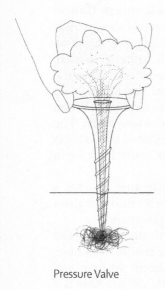

Pressure Valve

you have ultimate creativity at this level. You can do anything, and imagine anything you wish to help release the symptom, as long as you are willing to allow yourself to believe the story you are imagining.

You can use pressure valves to release pain, if you imagine that pain is an experience of energy not flowing freely, because of too much pressure inside which needs to be released. You can quickly release any kind of pain in this way, although headaches seem to be particularly easy to handle, no matter how long they have been there.

The pressure valve can look like a screw with a hole through it, which is screwed into the person in the place where the pressure is being felt. When the pressure valve reaches that place, you can then watch the pressure being released outward, with a *whoosh,* and the subject will feel the release at the same time. Both you and subject will experience the thought form as real, even though this time it began in your consciousness as the healer.

You should remember to remove the valve afterward, because you can use it again.

Thought forms can follow the description of how the subject experienced the symptom, as a thing, and then it is important that the healer work with that thing, since in the consciousness of the subject, it is that thing which stands between them and the experience of their wholeness.

The thought form can also be something the healer imagines that fits the description offered by the subject. For example, the healer can see knees that do not move freely as "rusty," and can use etheric oil to heal the subject. Thought forms can also be things imagined by the healer to help with the release of the symptom, as with the pressure valves.

If the healer knows anatomy or physiology, this too can be used, so that faulty or non-functional organs can be repaired. "Inflamed" muscles can have the flames put out. "Sleeping" organs can be awakened.

Working with thought forms also gives us possibilities of releasing people from dependencies, whether these have to do with substances, or ideas, or relationships. In cases of dependency or addiction, we say the subject is "hooked." When they do not get what they want, they feel bad, and the degree of bad that they feel shows how much they were hooked. When they feel bad, it feels bad in a particular place. When you look inside the subject in that place, then, you can see a hook and remove it. When the hook is removed, the subject is no longer hooked.

Obviously, this works when subjects sincerely wish to be released from the addiction. If they are not sincere, but rather just going along with what someone else wants for them, there will not be the same degree of success as with someone who has sincerely had enough of the addiction, and is ready to release it.

Even when the addiction was to a substance, the hook will show itself in one chakra or another. Remember that it is not the substance that is the problem, but rather the addictive personality, which is focusing on that substance. The hook will show itself at the location of the true addiction, which may actually be to security or power, etc., and which can then be released at that level.

While our orientation with the chakras involves a vertical model of wholeness, with individual balancing of the chakras along a vertical axis, some people have a need for a horizontal balancing. That is, there is an imbalance between their male side and their female side. This may manifest as one side of the body habitually experiencing symptoms or paralysis, or the two eyes not working together, or as dyslexia, where it is apparent that the two sides of the brain have not been "talking" to each other.

When the male brain and the female brain have not been talking, it usually represents the mother and the father not talking. If the parents experienced a strong non-harmonious polarity between them, it is easy to imagine how difficult it might have been for their children. In order to

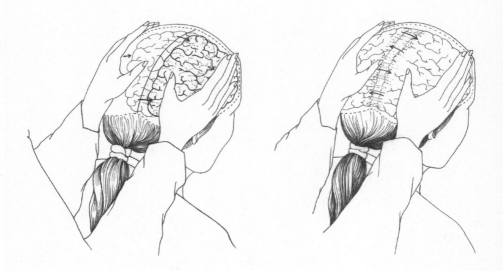

Psychic Brain Surgery

connect with one parent, they would have to disconnect with the other, and vice versa. It would be difficult for the child to be open to both energies at the same time.

To resolve the situation, we can do some quick brain surgery.

As the healer, you can look down at the subject's head, and imagine that you see the two halves of the brain. You can imagine one side of the brain entering the other, and staying there for a while, and then coming out again. Then you can repeat the process in the other direction.

When you have done this, each side of the brain has had a chance to experience the other, and there can then be a possibility for communication between them, where before there had been a wall of misunderstanding. Where the non-communication between the two halves of the brain had been the basis for a symptom, the conditions can now exist for the release of the symptom.

Some of the examples mentioned here may sound ridiculous, unbelievable, or like a joke, but they have all been used by healers, successfully. We believe that what one person can do, any other person can do, and that any being we see as extraordinary is merely showing us an example of our own capabilities. We believe that you, too, can use these tools successfully, to the degree you allow yourself to believe in them.

After all, whatever you believe to be true is true—for you.

Anything can be healed.

CHAPTER 10

Roots, Branches, and Crown

When you are experiencing your wellness, you are not only balanced at the level of the chakras, you are also integrated in terms of your connectedness with the earth, through the Red Chakra, and your openness to the cosmic energies we associate with the Violet Chakra.

During a healing, when the Red Chakra has been balanced, ask it to send roots down the subject's legs and into the earth, and watch to see what happens when you do this. The scene that presents itself to you shows you the subject's willingness to reach for nourishment from a valid source, just as a plant can send roots into the earth and reasonably expect its needs to be met in that way.

When the roots are reluctant to go down the legs, the subject is reluctant to reach outside themselves for the satisfaction of their needs, and this orientation towards self-sufficiency is neither necessary, nor useful. Of

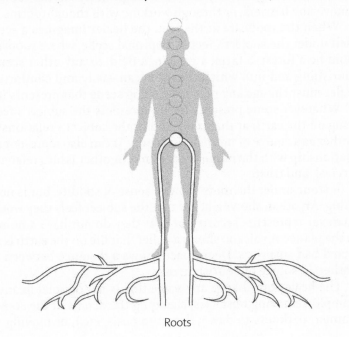

Roots

course, it is good to be self-sufficient when it is necessary, but if it is insisted on when unnecessary, it can be reflecting a reluctance based on previous experiences, a reluctance which does not serve the subject, but rather shows basic beliefs that if they do reach out, their needs will not be met.

Note: Healing is always about the subject's state of balance relative to who they are, and to where they are in their evolution. Thus, they would not show to their healer something needing to change unless their higher self, their inner being, wanted it to be seen. In any event, after the healing, both healer and subject will have the perception that whatever might have been a problem is one no longer.

If the reluctance is in both roots, right and left, it reflects basic beliefs about the general process of allowing oneself to be nourished. If it is only on the male side, it reflects non-trust in relation to reaching for nourishment from a male, and if on the female side, non-trust in relation to reaching for nourishment from a female.

If the blockage has been there for some time, it could reflect basic beliefs established in relation to the subject's mother or father, and if more recent, the healer and subject can examine the event in the subject's life corresponding to the onset of the symptom to see the applicability of the explanation. In any case, the healer should insist on encouraging the roots to proceed down the legs to the feet, removing any obstacles that present themselves along the way, either through watching the roots themselves remove any barriers, or through working with thought forms.

When the roots are at the feet, the healer imagines a scene showing itself under the subject's feet. An optimal scene, where roots enjoy being, could be a forest, a farm, a garden, a field, or any other scene with rich, nourishing soil into which the roots can easily and comfortably go. The healer must change any non-nourishing scene that presents itself.

Whatever scene presents itself represents the subject's feelings about being on the earth at that time, and/or the subject's relationship with the mother as a source of nourishing energy. It can also represent the subject's relationship with the home at that time, or other issues related to security, survival, and trust.

A stone under the roots shows a sense of solidity, but is not very nourishing. An ocean shows a belief that the subject feels they would drown in whatever represents security, or that they do not have a home anywhere on the planet. A volcano shows a belief that life on the earth is full of unexpected bad surprises. Deep space shows a distance between subject and mother, or source of nourishment.

The healer can change any scene that is not optimal in any way by, for example, removing obstacles, changing the details of the scene (winter to summer, darkness to dawn, desert to oasis, etc.), or moving the roots to another scene more welcoming to them (a graveyard to a park, bringing a boat to shore, changing the geographical location, etc.). When you as the healer do this, you have changed the image in the subject's consciousness that represented a belief system not working for them, into one that will result in success.

When the scene is optimal, you can ask the roots to enter the earth. Here, the image should optimally be that of a ball of nourishment in the center of the earth, clear red, which responds to the roots touching it by immediately being drawn up the roots toward the surface of the earth, up the legs, and into the Red Chakra of the person.

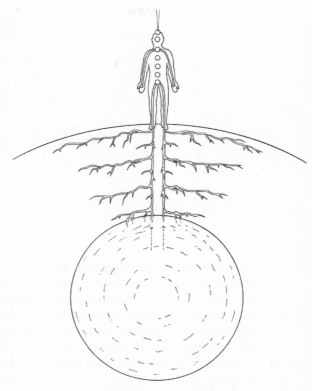

Taking Nourishment: Roots in Earth

This scene reflects (originally) the subject's beliefs about their mother as a source of nourishment, and (subsequently) the subject's relationship with sources of nourishment in general, whether about money, or about allowing their inner being to be nourished.

Again, if the scene is not optimal, you can change the scene, and when you do, the subject will experience a shift in consciousness, and, as often reported, a different sensation in the feet, feeling more contact with the earth, and being more present in the body.

Just as you ask the Red Chakra to put roots into the earth, you ask the Blue Chakra to put branches out through the arms. (The Blue Chakra is concerned with expressing.) When you do this, you can see the subject's beliefs and what is happening in their consciousness concerning expressing wants and feelings, and reaching for and having what they want, and what will make them happy.

The branches should not stop at the palms of the hands, but should continue beyond them, in the form of blue lasers, which meet at some

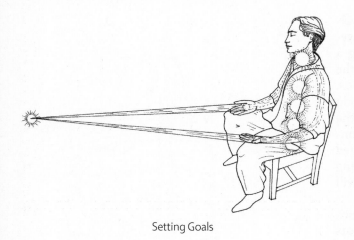

Setting Goals

distance in front of the subject. This shows the subject's ability to set goals, and what they believe will happen when they do that. The Blue Chakra, associated with the ether, the matrix on which reality is projected and the crossover between the physical and spiritual realities, represents their ability to manifest their goals, creating them in physical reality.

If the lasers do not extend beyond the palms, the subject does not bother setting goals important to them, because they do not believe they will happen anyway. The fact that this shows itself during the healing indicates that this is not a reflection of what is real and true for the subject, or what represents balance for them in terms of who they are, and where they are in their evolution. It needs to change.

If the beams do not focus on the same point, this is interpreted as the subject's desires not being what will make them happy. When this is the case, the healer aims the beams as they would the headlights of a car, until both beams focus on the same point. This should be at a distance that looks "right" to the healer. Closer in represents near goals, and farther out represents far goals. Optimally, the subject should have the flexibility to set goals at any distance.

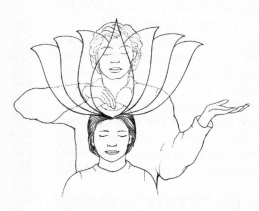

Healing the Violet Chakra

Watching the beams of energy flow down the arms will have a positive effect on symptoms that had affected the arms and shoulders, as watching the roots go down the legs will have a positive effect on symptoms that had affected the legs.

When the healer is working on the Violet Chakra, after it has been seen in its optimal state as a clear violet ball of energy, and while touching the top of the Violet Chakra, the healer asks the Violet Chakra to open, and watches what happens when it does that. Optimally, the Violet Chakra opens from the top, unfolding layer after layer of beautiful violet petals, like a lotus opening. If it does not do that, the healer needs to remove something that has been an obstacle there.

Since the Violet Chakra represents the deepest part of the subject's consciousness, when it is open, you can look through the Violet Chakra all the way down to the Red Chakra. When you can do this, you then ask White Light from above to enter the Violet Chakra, going all the way to the subject's toes, and then filling the subject from the toes up. As the White Light reaches each chakra, that chakra glows with the proper color, brighter and clearer than before. When the White Light overflows the Violet Chakra, it then surrounds the subject, as well as filling them, and the healer then knows that the healing is complete.

The final picture should be of the subject filled with White Light, with each chakra glowing brightly in its natural color, roots drawing nourishment from the center of the earth, blue lasers coming from the palms of the hands and meeting at some point in front of the subject, the subject's Crown Chakra opening like a lotus, and White Light continuing to flow into the subject and overflow around them. The subject should then be feeling quite different from how they felt before the healing. Just ask. And see the degree to which the healing has happened.

Anything can be healed.

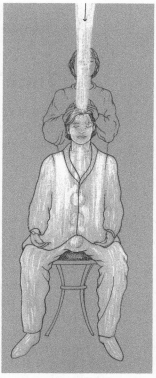

Healing the Violet Chakra—
Final Rinse

CHAPTER 11

Time Travel and Past Lives

Within our definition of consciousness, we identify three levels of being that we call soul, spirit, and personality. The soul is that part of you that travels through lifetime after lifetime, and that takes different forms within each lifetime, forms that we call spirit.

The spirit, then, is the individualized form that your consciousness takes within a certain lifetime, with individualized experiences and talents for the individualized purpose of that spirit which you are within that lifetime. The nature of consciousness is to move toward the completion of the pictures that represent the goals of that consciousness. When you have a goal, or a desire, the fulfillment of the desire exists, and you are moving toward that fulfillment. At the same time, apparently external events are bringing that fulfillment closer to you. In a particular lifetime, when circumstances present the opportunity to accept delivery of the experience you have asked for, there is always the option of agreeing to the delivery, or choosing to decline the offer. So, you go through life accepting or declining the experiences that had been the result of the pictures you had been putting in your consciousness, representing desires or goals you have had.

When you reach the end of a lifetime, and there are as yet unfulfilled goals, you have the opportunity to choose another lifetime which is designed to complete those unfulfilled goals, manifesting your soul in the form of another spirit. As you do this, and create more goals, the process continues until you have experienced everything you have asked for. Then, you go somewhere else and do something else in another universe. The process goes on forever. The only constant is change. Through change, we learn, and through learning, we grow. The nature of consciousness, which is what and who we are, is to grow, through learning, through change.

When you come into a human form, you are spirit manifesting, with a mind. As you learn things, and are rewarded for that with love, you identify yourself more and more by what you know, rather than by who you are, and you construct the sense of identity we call *personality*.

Sometimes, the personality and spirit are not aligned. They can pull in different directions, creating tension, and we can say that when that tension is healed, the healing happens at the level of the personality, by creating an alignment with spirit.

Each spirit has its sensitivities, and when the healing happens to the out-of-balance condition caused by these sensitivities having been touched, we can say that it happens at the level of the spirit.

It is said that the thought held at the moment of death stays with the being as they leave the body. The part of our consciousness that leaves a lifetime and chooses to enter another is what we have defined as the *soul*. Therefore, an out-of-balance condition carried over from another lifetime needs to be healed at the level of the soul.

Even though the condition resulted from tensions in a previous lifetime, those tensions have their correlation in this lifetime. For example, those who chose to come to earth to be healers several hundred years ago, at a time when it was not as widely accepted as it is now, may have found themselves persecuted, tortured, and killed for having chosen a life dedicated to helping others. For protection, these healers formed groups, rebelling against those portions of society that had oppressed them.

Western traditions teach that God is a Being outside ourselves who decides what will happen to us. Accordingly, these healers did not see that from the point of view that everything begins in our own consciousness, with the God within, it was they who had decided to come to earth with the mission of healing, and not God who had given them that assignment.

Many of them decided to be angry with God for having allowed this injustice, this persecution of beings that came to earth to help others, and they died with these thoughts in their consciousness. The result of that decision to be angry was to close the Violet Chakra, at the level of the soul. (It is the Violet Chakra that is concerned with the person's relationship with their father, with authority, and with God.)

When it was time to re-enter the earth plane, they then had to choose parents who would reflect the current state of imbalance within their energy systems, in order to heal the imbalance. So, they chose lives with fathers who were not there for them, or who could give them valid reasons for being angry. The healing, then, could come through the realization that everything in their experience does indeed begin within their own consciousness, or through the healing of their relationship with their father in this lifetime, or through a combination of the two.

We can see, then, that even though the original decision that created the imbalance was made in a previous lifetime, there were also real reasons in this lifetime to make the same decisions. When the healing happens in this lifetime, it then clears the effects of previous lifetimes, as well.

While exploring past lives may help us realize our immortal spiritual nature, it also can give us reasons to avoid facing current issues in our lives, and in that way, can be counterproductive to our evolution. If we continue to avoid issues in this way then our next lifetime will be a life full of tensions from our current life that still need to be released. It is only when knowledge of past lives helps us to resolve issues in our current life that it can be useful and helpful in terms of healing.

Since we are not limited by time or space, we can imagine ourselves traveling to these previous experiences in order to change something there, and then returning to this time frame, to see the positive effects of the healing.

One woman told me that in a previous life, she had been a member of European royalty, with a child, and that during one of the many wars of that period, the invading enemy took her child away. While she wanted to scream at the time, the scream never was released, because she was killed at that moment. She believed that it was because of this that she had had problems with her throat for her entire present lifetime.

During the healing, I saw the scene of the battle at the castle, with the soldier carrying away the baby, and another soldier preparing to throw a spear at the mother, to kill her. I blew some smoke in the eyes of the second soldier, so that there was a moment's hesitation before the spear was thrown. The scream came out, and after that, the mother was killed. It was, after all, her time to go, and she did not want to continue life without her baby. But she did have the chance to release the scream from her throat. After the healing, her throat was fine.

During another healing, I had an impression of the subject, an adult male, as a young boy whose father had just died. My first impulse was to pick up the child and hug him, to comfort him in some way, but that was not what he wanted or needed, so I just stood there, offering my hand. The boy took my hand and felt happy with that. We walked a bit, looking out in a certain direction. We were just aware of each other's presence, and very focused on what was being experienced, and the sense that it was being experienced together. Then, we walked a bit more and looked out in another direction, just being there together, in that experience. After that, we returned to the place from where we had started. That satisfied the boy, and the boy then quickly grew to the adult age of the man being healed.

The child had grown up in his life feeling incomplete that he had not the opportunity to share his experiences with his father, and when those experiences could be lived through the healing, he could then advance to the present with the consciousness of someone not having missed that experience. We could also say that his father's spirit was there for the healing, functioning through the healer.

When these scenes present themselves, they are subjective experiences, like watching and participating in mini-movies created by one's own active imagination. The interesting thing, of course, is that these imaginary movies are often experienced by both the healer and the subject, and also result in something being healed. When the paradigm, even when constructed, results in the release of symptoms, we must acknowledge it as having been a valid reality.

The important thing here is the realization that there are no limits to the healing process. While the healer may start the experience with no idea of traveling in time, the conditions encountered during the healing may be leading in that direction. If so, the healer can feel confident that whatever presents itself during the healing is part of the healing, and can respond in the moment of experience in the way that feels right during that moment.

Afterwards, we can look back at the apparent scenario that presented itself, and the effects of what we did, and be amazed by the play of consciousness, and the dimensions of healing, and what we have learned from it.

We can be amazed, that is, until we can consider it our new ordinary reality, and can then look forward to even more dimensions of consciousness and healing presenting themselves.

The process continues, infinitely.

It's something to do while we are here.

Anything can be healed.

CHAPTER 12

Levels of Experience

Each of the chakras not only represents a portion of your consciousness, but also is associated with one of the various bodies of which you are composed. It represents also a certain plane of consciousness, a level of experience from which you can see things differently, and a level of being, relative to the center of your being.

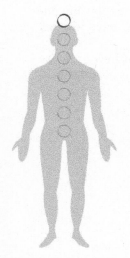

Violet Chakra—Causal Body
(Soul)

Thus, from the point of view of being a consciousness within a body, your deepest inner experience of yourself must be what we have described as a single point of consciousness glowing with intelligence, in the center of the Violet Chakra.

Being the deepest part of your consciousness, it is associated with the causal body, and the causal plane of consciousness, because if everything begins in your own consciousness, the deepest part of that consciousness representing your deepest desires and goals must be the cause of everything that happens. It is also a reflection of the idea that it is the home of God, and that God exists in you, as you, seeing the world through your eyes.

In a particular lifetime, the soul takes the form of an individualized consciousness that we call the spirit. It is like an overcoat that the soul wears in that lifetime, and therefore the next level of experience out from the center.

The spirit is associated with the Indigo Chakra and what is known as the Buddhic body and the Buddhic plane of consciousness. It is said to represent the level of perception experienced by Buddha and other beings who have reached the same level of awareness. Of course, we know that it also represents various levels of spirit-to-spirit communication, and the level from which we watch the outer manifestation of that which is going on within.

Following the same direction, the next level of experience out from the center must be the one associated with the Blue Chakra, which we associate with the element of the ether, the matrix on which physical reality is

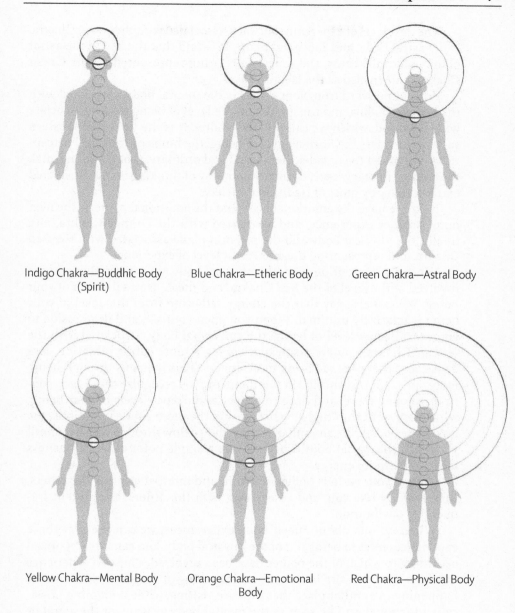

Indigo Chakra—Buddhic Body (Spirit)

Blue Chakra—Etheric Body

Green Chakra—Astral Body

Yellow Chakra—Mental Body

Orange Chakra—Emotional Body

Red Chakra—Physical Body

projected, the crossover between the physical and spiritual universes. It is called, of course, the etheric body, and the etheric plane of consciousness. It is the plane of manifestation in the physical world, and the place where thought forms exist.

The next level of experience outward, associated with the Green Chakra, is the astral body, and the astral plane. It is said that the key to the astral plane is harmlessness, the aspect of relating represented by the Green Chakra, known also as the Heart Chakra.

Further outward from your center is the mental body, associated with the Yellow Chakra, and the mind, and the level of being that we associate with the mind, which we call the personality. It is the level that Western society considers the normal level of being, the home of "normal" perceptions. We prefer to consider them usual and ordinary, though not normal. It would seem that what is normal for our way of thinking is still considered extraordinary by most of traditional society.

Next, we have the emotional body and the emotional plane as the next outer level of experience, and associated with the Orange Chakra, and finally, the physical body and the physical plane associated with the Red Chakra, and representing the outermost level of experience.

When your attention is on the physical body, we can say that you are involved at the level of the Red Chakra, and the densest vibration of your being. We can also say that the energy radiating from this level of your being is relatively minimal. When you open yourself, and drop inside to your next deeper level of being, the emotional body, associated with the Orange Chakra, you are also experiencing a more subtle vibration, less dense, and therefore radiating more energy. This happens through being more open. As you continue in this direction, you recognize that as you continue to open more, and drop to deeper and deeper levels of your being, which represent the "higher" chakras and the more subtle vibrations, the less dense bodies, the amount of energy able to flow through increases until you reach the causal body. Then you are a single point of consciousness radiating infinite energy.

Each of your various bodies is within and interpenetrating the others, each looking like you, and co-existing with the others, at different frequencies of vibration.

When we talk about out-of-body experiences, we can see that these experiences refer to being out of the physical body, and can be categorized according to which of the bodies have been involved. Thus, an experience in which a subject sits in one room, describing at the same time what is happening in another place that they are visiting, while remaining physically functional, can be seen as the mental body visiting, or the astral or etheric, depending on the apparent scenario being experienced.

Another kind of experience where our consciousness is present in another place while our body is non-functional can be described as our spirit traveling, and when we leave our body and do not return, we can describe that as the causal body, the soul, which has left.

An experience of fainting, or leaving the physical body during an epileptic fit, is a letting go at the level of the Red Chakra, which we associate with the physical body. In these cases, the person can be brought back into the physical body by re-establishing red in the Red Chakra, sending roots into the earth, and drawing the nourishment up from there into the legs, and then into the Red Chakra.

When your consciousness is in a particular chakra, we can say that you are occupying the body associated with that chakra, and seeing the world through that chakra can also be described as seeing from the plane of experience associated with that chakra.

Experiencing the different planes of experience is like being in different countries, where things happen in different ways, according to different principles. Cause-and-effect relationships are different.

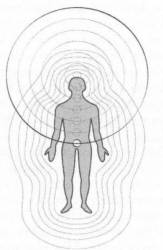

Auras & Levels of Experience, Physical

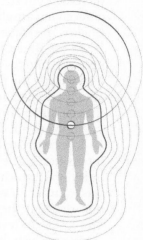

Auras & Levels of Experience, Emotional

At the level of the Yellow Chakra and below, we are concerned with ourselves and our needs, and physical cause-and-effect reality, as well as emotional needs and the pleasure principle, orienting ourselves toward that which feels best. At this level, things happen in a certain way. When you experience a certain lack, something that you want or do not have, there is a way to get it, but you must do something. You must work at it, or visualize, or use affirmations, but you must do to get. If you don't do, you don't get.

It is said that an aspect of the astral plane is harmlessness, and when looking at that countryside, it is apparent that everyone is expressing their love in their own way, and sometimes reacting to the perception that it is not there, until they can resolve their erroneous perception. It becomes apparent that love is the unifying force bringing us together, and the cosmic glue connecting everything in the universe. From this plane we see how our personal purposes can be served without causing harm to another. In fact, it is seen how satisfying someone else's needs can be the key to having our own needs met.

At the level of the Blue Chakra, things work in a different way than at the Yellow. You never have a perception of lack, because you perceive an abundant universe. You think of things, and they happen with no effort on your part at all. If you use effort, you place yourself in the Yellow Chakra, and that which was manifesting through the Blue Chakra then is no longer there. The effortless flow, the path of least resistance, and the appreciation of receiving are all keys to the state of abundance represented by the Blue Chakra. At that level, you have to not do, to get.

In the Blue Chakra, we experience perfection, and things happening perfectly, and that we are exactly where we are supposed to be at that time, with exactly the people we are supposed to be with, or alone exactly as we are supposed to be, and doing exactly what we are supposed to be doing in that moment. We can easily say, "I love where I am. I love whom I am with. I love what I am doing."

Life begins to take on the aspect of a dream, and the sense of perfection intensifies, at the level of the Indigo Chakra. We can identify ourselves as Spirit, that which we have been relating to as if it were not us, but which was wanting for us everything we really wanted for ourselves, carrying out our wishes at the same time we felt ourselves carrying out the wishes of Spirit. It is the level from which Jesus could say, "My Father and I are One."

We are also directly aware of the communication that exists between spirits, whether these spirits are also occupying physical form, or representing other entities, such as nature spirits, the spirit of a group consciousness like a country, or that of "inanimate" objects, such as automobiles, buildings, and machines.

We are aware of the dynamics of co-creation, the interplay between the spirits, and thus the manifestation in the physical world of what is in the consciousness. We see the relationship directly between what is inside our consciousness, and what is outside in the physical world, not only for ourselves, but for other creators as well.

At the level of the causal plane, and the point of view of the single consciousness creating all that it perceives as a movie played for its own interest, we see all that happens as the result of just our own consciousness. We can see everything that exists, and all that we are, as a part of just one single consciousness.

Oneness is not only a concept, but also a direct experience. It is evident that all is within, and that with the freedom we have to adopt any state of consciousness we choose, without limit, we have the capability of adopting the consciousness of another being, or a thing, or even God, and experiencing that consciousness as if it were our own, within ourselves. A direct experience of meaning comes to the words, "We are I am."

We can experience ourselves as a single consciousness creating a dream, and experiencing that all of creation is the manifestation of that dream. We can be aware that we are dreaming within that dream, as we do in a lucid dream, and then deciding all that will happen within that dream, without limits.

We can dream that bones can mend, tumors dissolve, lame people can walk, blind people can really see. In a dream, there are no rules. We can dream whatever we wish. We can dream that we have unlimited abilities to heal whatever presents itself to be healed, know-

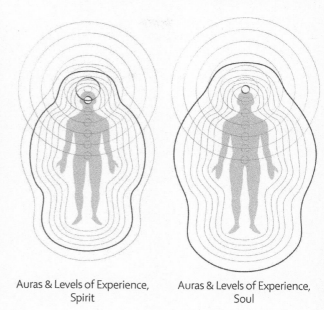

Auras & Levels of Experience, Spirit

Auras & Levels of Experience, Soul

ing that within the dream we are dreaming, within the scenario we are creating in our own consciousness, within the reality we are creating with our own perceptions in our own dream, *anything can be healed*.

How to Do It
Creation and Co-Creation

CHAPTER 13

Receiving Your Healing

There's a story about a woman who had cancer, and who had been told by her doctors that she had two weeks to live. She went to see the psychic surgeons in the Philippines, who performed the healing, and told her that she was healed. She didn't believe them, so two weeks later, she died. At her autopsy, however, the doctors found no cancer within her.

For each of us, our perceptions create our reality. This is, of course, as true for the person being healed, the subject, as it is for the healer. When we look at healing as a process of co-creation, we can see that there is a possibility for the subject to either interfere with the healing process or create an optimal environment in their consciousness in which the healing can happen. In the next two chapters, we will examine the perceptions on the part of the subject, the person being healed, which encourage the process of healing, and increase the probability and degree of success. In these chapters you will be asked to experience the healing process though the eyes of the subject, the person being healed.

When we are discussing perceptions, we are talking about what you, the subject, choose to think or feel, and how you choose to interpret events. As we all know by now, there is always a choice.

The person being healed can either passively allow the healing to happen, or actively encourage the process. It is not necessary to actually believe in what is happening, or in the structure of the healer's reality, but just to not get in the way of it. The important thing is to leave a door open for positive possibilities. You can say, for example, "Well, I have nothing to lose by going for it, and perhaps something positive can happen. Even though I don't understand it, it might help." Then you are passive and open and receptive to the healing.

To take a more active role, you can encourage the perception that your healing is happening *now*.

1. Preliminaries

During the interaction between the healer and the subject, the optimal environment is created when it is the subject who asks for the healing. Sometimes, well-intentioned friends or relatives ask the healer, on behalf of the subject, for the healing. This does not always reflect the intention or desire of the subject. Sometimes, the subject has not acknowledged that a healing is necessary, or is not comfortable for some reason with entering into the process of working with a healer. This must be respected.

Healing someone who does not want to be healed is like teaching a pig how to whistle. It is a waste of time, and it annoys the pig.

When a subject asks for a healing, it can be they who initiate the interaction, or they can respond to the healer's offer of help. If you are not feeling well and a healer asks "What can I do for you?" or "I'm a healer. Can I help you?" you may respond by expressing a desire to be healed. Or, you may yourself seek the healer, and ask for a healing.

The expressed desire to be healed should ideally be explicit, and not just implied. It's like a contract between the healer and the subject to do something that satisfies the subject's needs. The more explicit the words, the clearer the subject is that this thing going on in their body and/or consciousness needs to change. If you have hemorrhoids, for example, you should say so, and not "Well, I've got a little problem with my Red Chakra." If you have AIDS, you should say so, expressing a desire to heal that, expecting it to happen. It is, in other words, usually most effective for the subject to tell the healer exactly what it is that needs to be healed, and to do that as openly, as directly, and as clearly and briefly as possible.

The words, "I want to be healed," imply that a healing is needed. You are acknowledging that something has not been working for you as you would like it to, in your body and/or your life, and you have accepted that those are the conditions of the moment before the healing. You are also acknowledging that the healing is wanted, that you want the situation to change, and that you are ready to have the change happen now.

You are also saying that you expect it to happen *now*. It is for the healer to agree to the subject's request for a healing, also expecting it to happen, and in that action, to create an agreement of goals, an alignment of intentions in the consciousness of the beings taking part in that event.

When that is done, it is as though a movie has just begun, where the ending is known. The end of the movie is that the healing has happened. It just has not yet been acted through. It's a bit like seeing a James Bond movie. Before you sit down, you know the ending. The good guys win, the bad guys lose, the world is saved, and James Bond and the beautiful women find each other (usually, in a boat).

It's always the same, and yet we sit down, interested in how it happens this time. Healing works a bit like that, too. The ending has been defined, the healing has happened in the future, and all that remains is to act it through, watching it manifest in physical external reality. The intention has been set. With the preliminaries thus taken care of, the actual form of the healing may proceed.

Different healers use different forms of healing. Some prefer to work with the subject lying or sitting, so that the subject remains relaxed and open. Obviously, healing can happen with the subject in any particular prescribed position. If there is an accident, with a healer on the scene, it may not be appropriate for the healer to decide that before they can work on this situation the injured person must be on a table or chair, with soft lights, incense and music, and everyone being quiet. Aside from such cases of first aid, however, healers each decide for themselves a way of working that is optimal for them.

The preferred position within the Body Mirror System is for the subject to be seated in a chair which has an opening in the back that allows the healer to access the subject's back and base of the spine. We find that in this way, we are able to reach virtually every part of the subject's body.

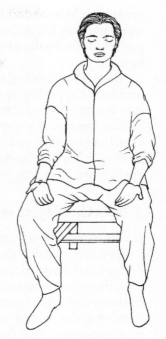

Open for the Healing

The subject sits with feet flat on the floor, hands in lap with the palms facing upward, and with the eyes closed. This is a physical position that reflects the inner posture of openness and positive expectancy. The eyes are closed to allow the subject to keep their attention on merely being present and open for the healing. They open their consciousness to the healer, allowing themselves to be totally visible. A desire to hide a part of their consciousness from the healer reflects a decision to not heal that part of their consciousness, or to not experience wholeness in that part of their consciousness. Total openness is most effective.

2. Subject's perceptions of the healer

It would not make sense for you, when you are the subject, to hold the perception that this healer does not really know what they are doing, or that they will not do a good job. That's not the reality you should wish to create with your perceptions, nor with the words you are using in speaking to yourself describing the experience you are entering. Your most intelligent option would be to decide that this healer might be the greatest healer the world has ever known, whether that healer knows it or not, and absolutely perfect for the healing that needs to happen, and which is, in fact, about to happen.

During the healing, you should continue to remind yourself that your healing is happening *now,* and that the perfect healer for you is doing whatever is necessary to achieve that. I know of no healers who need the subject to help them in any way during the healing. It is not necessary for you to visualize anything, or hold a thought on anything other than "My perfect healing is happening *now."* After all, if the greatest healer the world has ever known is healing you, they certainly do not need your help. Right?

3. Does the subject really expect to be healed?

If you, as the subject, are looking forward to another healing that is to happen after the one that you are receiving *now,* you are not expecting to be healed during *this* healing. When someone really wants to be healed, then they want to be healed *now.* To agree, before the healing, to a series of healings that will be necessary to solve the problem is also to decide beforehand that the healing will not be complete this time. We prefer to work with conditions that can create the one-visit healing. Potentially, that is what is possible.

After the full effects of the healing have been experienced, which might be up to two weeks after the act of the healing, it can be seen whether the effects were partial or total, and if partial, another healing can be arranged, but again, with the expectancy that *this time,* the effects will be total. If a subject is looking forward to working with another healer after the one that is working with them now, they are also not expecting to be healed during this healing.

If a subject is wearing eyeglasses or a hearing aid during the healing, that implies that they expect to need them after the healing, and to that degree, they do not really expect the total healing to happen.

When you are the subject, you should be anticipating that when the healing is complete something will be different, and be eager to see, in that moment after the healing, what your experience shows you about the effects of the healing you have had.

4. Completing the healing

When you open your eyes after having received a healing, your first thoughts should be that the healing has happened. You can take an immediate personal inventory of the way you feel in your body, in your consciousness, and in any senses or functions that had been impaired before, and notice how you feel now compared to how you felt before. Your first thoughts should be directed to what is different, in a way that is recognized as better, even if it is just, "more relaxed."

With each acknowledged improvement, others become evident. It is as if you are entering the new bubble, deeper and deeper, with each recognition of the positive effects of the healing. Even improvements that are only partial should be acknowledged, indicating the degree of improvement noticed so far. There should also be the understanding that whatever improvement has been noticed immediately is likely to continue, and that more effects will be noticed afterwards. After the positive feedback, you can communicate to the healer any symptoms that remain to be released. Often, the healer will agree to then complete the healing, aligning their perceptions with your feedback, seeing the degree to which the remaining symptoms are ready to be released.

For example, you might say, "My knee feels better than before, but not yet completely healed. It feels like 30% of the discomfort remains from what was there before." The healer can then go directly to the place where the discomfort remains, and do what they can to quickly release it. If it releases quickly, the process is complete. Otherwise, the healer can proceed with giving you the feedback, as described in the next chapter, giving the remaining symptoms time to release further. Often, after the feedback, the remaining symptoms are gone, but if not, the healer can then quickly release whatever is left.

With your verbal acknowledgment of the healing, and of the positive effects of the healing, you can then maintain your attention in the present moment, with a more positive view of the future than you had before. Events in the physical world that are clearly improvements over what had been there before will then solidify this view, and make it more and more evident that your healing has happened.

5. After the healing

During a healing, the healer must create the expectancy that the effects of the healing will be immediate, but they must also know how to look at the situation when the full effects may not yet be immediately apparent, while holding the perception that the healing has happened. In this way, you, the subject, the person who has been healed, can also maintain a positive sense of expectancy for continuing effects.

In a healing, both healer and subject are working at deep levels of consciousness. The effects of the healing must move through their different levels of experience, their different levels of consciousness, until they are fully manifest on the physical level. This takes time, but the amount of time that it takes may be variable. For some people, the complete manifestation of the healing may take a matter of minutes. For others, it may take hours, days, or weeks, depending on the sensitivities of the subject, and their beliefs about what is possible. Normally, we can expect the full effects of the healing to have manifested totally anywhere between three days and two weeks after the act of the healing.

The deepest inner experience of which you are capable is at the level that we call the soul, associated with the Violet Chakra. Your outermost level of experience, at the level of the physical body, is associated with the Red Chakra. Between the two are the remaining levels of experience that we associate with different levels of consciousness, the different subtle bodies, and the different chakras.

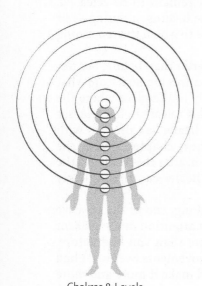

During the time it takes for the full effects of your healing to manifest, the effects ripple through the different levels of your consciousness, and you experience the corresponding changes in your consciousness as changes in your way of thinking. New ideas are able to come in and make sense of things in a new way, releasing old tensions that had been associated with the old ideas.

You are then able to examine your interactions in the world around you, the way you choose to respond to conditions, and notice those that are different from before, recognizing the process as the continuing effects of the healing that you had received.

Chakras & Levels
of Experience

You, the subject, may experience sensations as if things are moving in your body, as the physical structure rearranges itself to come into balance with the new configuration of energy, until the full effects of the healing have been experienced. If, after two weeks, any traces of the symptoms remain, you can accept the degree of the healing that has happened so far, and prepare yourself to release the rest. Then, when the healing is complete, you can get on with your life, busying yourself with other priorities, like living your dreams, and finding happiness in your own way. You are healed, and there is nothing further to do about that.

Healed is healed.

Anything can be healed.

CHAPTER 14

Accepting Your Healing
(Healing and Transformation)

Each type of illness is associated with a particular way of being. There is a personality type associated with heart disease; there is another associated with cancer; another with nearsightedness, etc. The person's way of being has had stress associated with it, and that stress has reached the physical level, manifesting as a symptom.

When someone wants to release a symptom, they must release the way of being that was associated with the symptom, and which, in fact, created it. Releasing the stress from the consciousness allows them to then have different perceptions, and a different way of being. There is a change in the nature of the bubble, the filter of perceptions through which they see the world. Said another way, since our perceptions create our reality, there is a change or movement from one bubble to another, from one reality to another, from one paradigm to another.

Thus, we can say that the process of healing implies a process of transformation. In the experience of this writer, recovery from catastrophic illness is always accompanied by a change in the person's way of being. They change, or else continue to manifest the symptoms until they die. Those who change are able to see things differently in their lives, and to notice that things happen in ways different from before. They are able, through having different experiences, to define different beliefs. Or, they are able to first define different beliefs, and then have different experiences.

The important thing, in either case, is to release old perceptions that have been based on old experiences, if those perceptions have resulted in a tense way of interacting with the environment.

One way to achieve this reprogramming, this perception modification, is by recognizing the element of time as a possible distorting influence in our internal programs and perceptions, and by choosing to not prejudice our positive view of the present and future by our negative experience of the past.

For example, you might have a program in your human biocomputer that says, "Every time I see Jill, I get a headache!" Then, given Jill, the headache is expected, so that you have a chance to affirm that truth, the program that is believed to be true, and therefore, is true for you. Unfortunately, the program always results in a headache, so although the program is very effective and efficient, the result is something unpleasant.

To release the program while still acknowledging what is true, you can describe it as having been true in the past. Then, the program would say, "Every time that I *have seen* Jill, I *have gotten* a headache—but the next time might be different. Perhaps Jill has realized the error of her ways, or has become enlightened, or transformed (it's always a change in the other person). For the next time, I'll see what happens and what is true then."

Then, direct experience can show that something different is, in fact, true. "Wow! Jill really is different—and, actually, quite pleasant to be around! I'm sure I will never again get a headache from being around Jill." From that moment, with those words, a new belief is created, and new perceptions are allowed, and a new reality is created with the new belief.

If you are interested in experiencing the process of healing, and therefore, the process of transformation, what is particularly important is the way you describe yourself to yourself. This is because the words that you use to describe your experience create your reality, and you are interested in the creation of a different reality in which you feel better than you did before.

Thus, it's important to pay attention to the words that you use to describe yourself. If you are describing some trait you do not find particularly successful ("I'm shy," or "I'm afraid of success," or "I'm naturally irritable," etc.), then with your words, leave it in the past, making room for a different perception in the present, and also the future ("I *was* shy," or "I *have been* afraid of success," or "I was irritable because I was not really being myself," etc.).

In that way, you will be able to more easily dis-identify with and therefore let go of old ideas, and old tensions associated with the symptoms to be released.

The same is true about the words you use to describe the symptom to be released. Consider the element of time, and be able to describe the symptom to yourself as you experience it in the present moment. If you say, "It hurts all day," you may not be noticing that, in fact, it doesn't hurt so much right now. If you say, "The symptom comes and goes," when you do not experience it right now, you expect it to return. It is more effective to describe your experience in the present moment, acknowledging what is true now, and with a positive orientation toward a positive future ("It's better now than it has been. In fact, it really seems to be getting better and better.").

The positive mental attitude is, of course, an element useful for enjoying the best quality of life achievable. For the process of healing, however, it is essential.

Whatever you visualize, you improve the probability of happening. The images or pictures that you put into your consciousness have more of a tendency to happen. If you continue to put into your consciousness pictures of yourself suffering, you tend to continue that condition. It does not even matter what emotion you have with the picture—it is the picture that is important. Thus, if you have a picture of what you *do not* want, you are still having a tendency to fill your consciousness with that picture, and therefore, to create what you do not want.

It is important, then, to have in your consciousness a picture of the final positive result that you are working toward, as a reminder of your goal. When you are receiving a healing, optimally it should be with the expectancy of being healed. At the very least, it must not be with disbelief and resistance, which stop the process.

You do not have to believe in the method or system, but you must remain open to the possibility of it working for you. If you do believe in the healing, then during the healing you can remind yourself that your healing is happening *now*. After the healing has happened, you can see whether the results are partial or total, so far. Sometimes, the full effects of the healing are immediately apparent, although often there are continuing positive effects that manifest during the days or weeks following the healing act.

When the healing is total, and no symptoms are experienced, know that you are healed, and just get on with the rest of your life. When the full effects of the healing have not yet been experienced, it is important to continue to remind yourself that the healing has happened, and that the effects are on the way. Rather than continuing to see yourself in your old bubble, see yourself in your new bubble, the one you are moving toward. See yourself healed, in the future.

In changing your bubble, or moving from any one reality to any other, there are three steps:

1. Decide what will be true in the new reality

For example, you can decide, "In the new reality, when the healing is complete, the pain will be gone," or "Reading will be easier," or "The tumor will be gone."

2. Encourage the perception that it's happening now

While it's true that you are moving toward some goal in the future, and holding the perception of success at some point in the future, the process of reinforcement must happen in the present moment. The idea is to examine your perceptions of what is happening now, in the moment of experience: "The pain now is less than it was before. The healing must be happening now," or "The letters I see are a bit clearer now than before," or "Perhaps the tumor is actually a bit smaller now. Anyway, my consciousness feels more clear now, so I know that something positive is happening."

Positive thinking is not self-deception. Even when there are highs and lows in the experience of the symptoms, it's important to see that the lows are where the highs used to be, so that even on your current worst days, you feel better than you used to feel on your previous best days. In other words, even on days when the symptoms are being experienced, it can be noticed that they are not so severe as before (when that is true), and you are thus able to hold a perception of a positive direction.

The idea is to give yourself reasons to believe in the process, while at the same time, acknowledging what is true, on the physical level. It is, after all, the measurement on the physical level that shows the effects of the work being done in the consciousness. Each improvement in the condition on the physical level should be acknowledged, and owned, as evidence that the healing is happening now.

If the conditions on the physical level have been measured as continuing to deteriorate, it must be clear that something has not been working, so that steps can be taken to correct the situation, and continue the healing process. Even this necessary correction can be seen as part of the healing, and in fact, it is. It brings you one step closer to the final result of being healed.

3. Decide and know that *now*, it's true

You continue the encouragement process until you experience yourself symptom-free. When that happens, you must consider the possibility that you may never again experience that symptom. When the pain is gone, it may be gone for good. When you see clearly, you accept it as your new normal state. When the healing is complete, you must see yourself as healed, and in that way, we say that you own the healing. You identify the state of consciousness you experience, and your view of the world from that state of consciousness, as normal and usual for you, even if it is your *new* normal way of being.

If the symptom was evidenced on the basis of medical tests, look forward to new tests that show you as free of those symptoms. After all, healed is healed, and on all levels. If the tests show improvement, but not yet total results, know that you are moving in a positive direction, and that there is still a bit further to go. If you have been working on yourself, continue, accepting the progress you have made thus far. If you have been working with others healing you, you can know that it was a partial healing, and that the next one can take you further along, or be the one that is the last you will ever need.

When you have the feedback on the physical level that shows the effects of the healing work you have been doing, accept it and trust it, and when you have a clean bill of health, find other things to do with your consciousness than correcting problems. Get creative, and set goals, watching them manifest, creating with the tools you have learned to use, a life in which you are happy and fulfilled.

In fact, you may consider sharing your success story with others. Many healers and teachers of healing have started on this path through the necessity of healing themselves. Thus, when they share their stories, it is from their personal experience. That was the way it worked for me. Perhaps it can work that way for you, too.

Let everyone know that anything can be healed.

CHAPTER 15

Feedback

There is always an inner cause to each symptom. There is something that the subject has been doing in their consciousness that has resulted in the manifestation of the symptom. When the subject is healed, and thus returned to the experience of wholeness, they are once more in the state of consciousness in which they are clear.

The subject's experience of this may be that they feel somehow different, yet without a clear idea of exactly what is different. The tensions have been released, and there is a new way of seeing things, but until the subject examines the issues that had been seen before with tension, they may not be aware of the new view.

To that degree that subjects choose to make decisions and see things in the old way, out of habit, or to hold on to old ideas, they will be able to re-create the symptoms. To the degree that they stay in the new clear consciousness, they will continue to see things in the new way, and be able to remain symptom-free.

It is helpful, then, to let the subject know which areas of their consciousness have been cleared, and which specific ways of thinking had been associated with the symptom that had needed to be healed. In that way, they can consciously choose to do something different, knowing that it is for their own health and happiness.

It is a bit like taking your automobile to the mechanic for the same old problem it has been having for so long that has been fixed over and over again. If the mechanic tells you why the problem had been there, perhaps because of a certain habit while driving, you will know afterwards that to continue to have that habit will result in recurrence of the same problem, and that to do something different will mean to not have that problem any more.

Thus, an important element in the healing is the feedback, telling the subject the relationship between what had been happening in their consciousness, and what had been happening in their body, or the relationship between certain basic beliefs and the way things have happened in their life. The feedback takes place after the healing has happened. You, the healer, tell the subject what you saw, and what you did, and what it all means to you, with the intention of helping the subject re-orient themselves to the new bubble in which they are more clear, and healed, and know it. You communicate what thought forms you saw and removed, and what they represented to you. If there is no meaning to you, there should be one for the subject.

The things that are seen must make sense to at least one of the two participants in the healing, or those images would not have presented themselves. Sometimes, however, the meaning is realized only after some time. Of course, you never change the picture on the basis of whether the subject accepts the feedback or not. After all, what was seen was seen. The only variable can be the interpretation. If the interpretation is not clear, you can just feel satisfied to communicate the picture that was seen. If you were working with the chakras, you can communicate what you saw there, and what your interpretation is of what you saw, according to the Language of the Colors (Appendix 2). For example, you might say, "There was blue in your Red Chakra. That told me that you had been hungry for security. I removed the blue, and made it red. You should be feeling more of a sense of solidity now, and you can look forward to more of a sense of satisfaction of your security needs, such as your relationship with money."

The subject might respond, "It was since my mother died that all of these other things became problems. Now, I can see the connection. Also, I no longer feel the same sense of missing her, but rather just loving what she has been for me in my life, and feeling the need to get on with my life. Anyway, I still feel surrounded with her love, and that feels great." Thus, it should be clear that the feedback does not represent something that is still a problem, but rather is about the problem that was there before the healing, which has been released, and about the positive results the subject can look forward to after the healing.

Here's another example: you might say, "I saw a kind of shell around your Solar Plexus Chakra and released it. It was as if you had felt closed-in before, and now there should be more of a sense of ease." A response from the subject might be, "Yes, that talks to me. I had been feeling like that concerning circumstances in my life, and now I seem to feel more of a sense of space. Thank you."

If you say, "You had not been letting yourself be nourished. It probably started with your relationship with your mother," the subject might leave with the impression that they still have a problem with their mother, and that it is because their mother did something wrong. They may also continue to have the impression that they have a problem with letting themselves be nourished, and will find reasons to continue to affirm the problem.

If, however, you add, "Now, it will be easier for you, and will feel natural for you, to nourish the inner being, and in addition, you can look forward to a new harmony in your relationship with your mother, and much more ease in letting in her love," the subject can leave with a positive sense of expectancy within the new reality, and with the perception of having been healed.

We could say that the feedback is not always necessary, since we are always in touch with our inner voice, and somewhere inside we know everything. That is true, of course, but then, hearing it again from the outside strengthens the message. Sometimes, the message has already been understood by the subject, and it has been only old beliefs, for example, not finding a way to believe how the symptom can be released, that have been holding on to the symptom. Then, the healing is the "excuse" the subject uses to release the symptom, and they have already gotten the message and applied it to what needs to be different in their lives in order for them to be happy.

When you provide the feedback to the subject, you are not telling them something they do not already know. Something inside them resonates with what you are saying. They recognize the validity of the communication. If not, they should let you know that.

When you are giving feedback, the subject can respond in one of two ways. Either they can say, "That talks to me," meaning that they recognize the validity of the feedback in terms of what they know to have been true about themselves, or, "I don't have an experience of that, but thank you for the feedback," meaning that at least for the moment, they do not identify with the feedback, but may recognize it some time later.

Another possibility, of course, is that the feedback does not fit the subject, and is an erroneous interpretation on your part. When you see things, the picture may be very clear, but perhaps not the interpretation. If this is the case, you and the subject both benefit from the subject saying that the feedback does not fit. Then, together you might find a much more fitting interpretation of the pictures that you saw.

It is, of course, in your interest to be as clear as possible regarding feedback, in order to be as effective as possible. After all, if you are going to do something, you might as well be as good at it as possible. If the subject tells you, "I don't have an experience of that," you must examine the nature of your own perceptions, and consider that you may have been interpreting the pictures you saw on the basis of your own bubble, and not that of the subject. If so, you can then make the necessary adjustment to the feedback, and to your own perceptions.

In the role of a healer, you must examine the anticipated effects of the communication with the subject, and whether it leaves the subject with the final impression of something having been healed, or of a problem remaining that had not been previously perceived. To tell someone, "Watch out for that woman with the red hat. She is not your friend," or, "I see an accident involving a car," only serves to plant the seeds of fear, doubt, and suspicion in the subject's consciousness, as well as a sense of dependency on the perceptions of the healer.

It would be more in the interests of the subject for you to leave them with a sense of trust in their own perceptions, and in their own ability to create a positive life for themselves without any further help from you. That, therefore, should be your orientation in providing the feedback, and in reinforcing the perception (your own, as well as the subject's) that the subject is now healed.

Our perceptions create our reality.

Anything can be healed.

CHAPTER 16

Healing Others—Preliminaries

Since our perceptions create our reality, you must create the perception in yourself that the subject is healed. There are several ways to achieve this perception.

One way to create the perception that the subject is healed is to use a model of wellness, or wholeness. With the tools we have discussed in this book, you have three possibilities, which are chakras, White Light, and thought forms. No matter which tools are used, however, it should be remembered that they are most effective when used with a positive sense of expectancy.

The person being healed is creating you as the healer with their perceptions. It is important when you are the healer that you play the part, if only for the short period of time that the healing requires. After that, you can allow yourself to be amazed at the miraculous results you have created, until you are able to see it as your new ordinary reality.

In the interaction between healer and subject immediately prior to the healing, either the subject will approach you and ask for something to be healed, or you will offer your services and the subject will respond by asking for something to be healed.

When you agree implicitly or explicitly to participate in the healing, you agree to align with the intentions of the subject. In that, you are yin to the subject's yang. That which establishes direction is what we define as *yang,* and that which agrees to support that direction and follow it, we define as *yin.*

After that, during the healing, it is you as the healer who is yang and who establishes the procedures, and the subject who agrees to be open and receptive, yin, in order to have their own needs met, as they have defined them before.

You as the healer do not ask the subject how the healing should proceed, nor do you follow the instructions of the subject. If you do that, you are leaving the process in the hands of the subject. Considering that the healing is happening in the perceptions of the healer, you as the healer must direct the activities during the healing. This can, of course, be done with consideration for the sensitivities of the subject, but it is still you as the healer who is creating the healing, with the subject agreeing to the perception. If the subject does not have confidence in your techniques as the healer, or does not agree with these techniques, they should stop the process, and seek their healing another way, or with another healer.

There is always another way.

The functions and perceptions of the healer can be placed in two categories of healing: classic healing and healing as first aid. Classic healing establishes optimal conditions for the healing, but with the understanding that these conditions are not necessarily prerequisites. If these conditions are not there, you can function as a healer anyway, as you must if first aid is called for. Even under these circumstances, you must maintain the perception that the healing is happening.

At the same time that we say the optimal healing is encouraged by a setting of soft lights and music, for example, you know that if ever you need to, you can perform a healing in Times Square with the traffic blaring, and the Rolling Stones singing *Brown Sugar* right next to you. As a healer, you must always maintain the perception that the healing is happening and is being effective.

No matter what the form of the healing, classic or first aid, using chakras, White Light, or thought forms, you always prepare yourself in the same way, by placing yourself in a state of consciousness in which you feel energy, and in which a healing can happen. This is described in Section V, "Basic Energy Exercises—Feeling Energy and Directing Energy." Your knowledge of preliminaries to the healing would not be complete without having read this material, and having done the exercises.

After having done these exercises, you will be prepared to better understand and follow the procedures described in the chapters that follow this one, so please take the time to do these exercises now.

Always, as a final step in preparing for the healing in which you are about to participate, remind yourself that you are never presented with a healing you are not capable of doing.

Anything can be healed.

CHAPTER 17

Healing with White Light

Here, you as the healer will use White Light as the model of wholeness, or wellness, to create the perception that the healing has happened. When you have imagined that the subject is filled with White Light, this will trigger the perception that the subject is healed.

White Light is used for healing because of all of its positive associations with purity and spirituality. In addition, White Light represents wholeness because it contains all of the colors of the spectrum. Wholeness is wellness.

When we think of a fluorescent tube, we see that when the energy flows through the tube, it glows. Then, White Light can also represent energy flowing freely, which fits well with our definition of healing as returning to the experience of wellness through release of blockages.

If White Light represents energy flowing freely, then energy not flowing freely is represented as shadows. When the subject is being filled with White Light, if shadows are seen, you should know that these simply represent tensions, and that more White Light should be shone on them. When light meets shadow, all that remains is light. The tensions were those that existed either in the consciousness or the physical body, or both. The shadows dissolving show the tensions dissolving.

Of course, then, if you feel tensions in the subject's body (in the shoulders, for example), or you know that there are tensions within the subject's body, you will also know that when you look inside, you are going to see the tensions as shadows. If you do not, you must adjust your perceptions until they are in accord with what you know to be true on the physical level. Then, starting with that, the shadows can be dissolved and the tensions released, and the healing can manifest.

In the classic White Light healing, see that the subject is seated comfortably, feet flat on the floor, hands open and relaxed in the lap, and eyes closed. Naturally, the subject will not be wearing eyeglasses or other prosthetic devices. Then, seeing that the subject is open and ready for their healing, you can begin with the Healing Starting Position, as described in Section V.

Feeling the energy in your hands, you know that you are in the ideal state of consciousness in which to feel energy, and in which a healing can

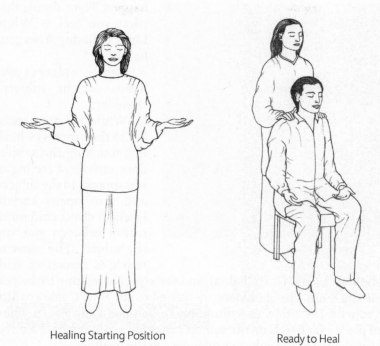

Healing Starting Position

Ready to Heal

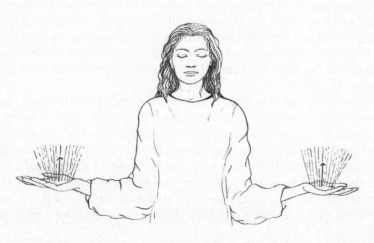

Healing Starting Position

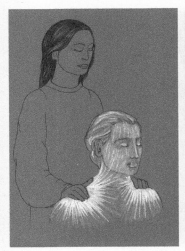
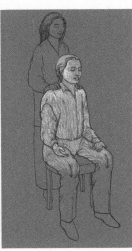

Filling the Subject

happen. Then, decide that what you feel is White Light radiating from your hands.

Gently place your hands on the subject's shoulders.

While it is not necessary to the process of healing, touching the subject does provide a feeling of reassurance to the subject, and also opens certain levels of direct communication between you and the subject. The sense of touch, is associated with the Green Chakra (the Heart Chakra), and the aspect of relating to the person inside the body. The shoulders are related to the Blue Chakra, which is involved with the subject's willingness to be open and receive. Thus, when you place your hands on the subject's shoulders, you can have a direct sense of the degree of the subject's openness to the healing.

It is emphasized here that the touch is light, and that there is no pressure, and no physical manipulation involved in this type of healing.

When your hands are glowing with White Light, imagine that you are filling the subject with this light, through the shoulders, up into the head, and then down through the body to the toes, also filling the body and the arms out to the skin. This can all be done with your hands resting on the subject's shoulders.

If you sense that it is difficult to enter the body and (therefore) the consciousness of the subject, communicate this silently, spirit to spirit, to the subject. It is like an imaginary conversation which says something like, "I'm here for your healing, but I'm having difficulty coming inside. Will you please open so that I can help you in the way I know how?" Usually, after that, the flow is easier. If it isn't, make the communication aloud. If there is still resistance, acknowledge that, and let the subject know that they need to work with another healer, or in another way, or at another time.

Imagine yourself filling the subject with White Light, in any way you choose. You might imagine a white substance flowing from your hands, filling the subject. Or, you might imagine that the subject is filled with millions of tiny fluorescent tubes, and that as the energy from your hands touches the tubes in a particular part of the body, that part glows.

If while placing your hands on the shoulders of the subject, you feel that the muscles are tense, you will know that when you look that you will see shadows. After all, shadows are tensions. You do not need to massage the subject's shoulders, but rather just shine White Light from your hands, watching the White Light melt the shadows as a heat lamp melts ice. When you do that, you will feel the subject's shoulders relax under your hands, on their own, without your exerting pressure.

As the subject is being filled with White Light, if you imagine that you see shadows, and dissolve them with light, remember where these shadows were perceived. You can then communicate this information to the subject in the form of feedback after the healing, thus letting the subject know where perceived tensions had been released.

When you see the subject totally filled with and glowing with this White Light, you have created the perception that the healing has happened. At that point, the healing is complete, and you should communicate that aloud to the subject, saying, "You can open your eyes when you like," and then wait for the subject's response.

You have created the perception that the healing has happened, and now need to know the degree to which the subject agrees with this perception. You can find this out by asking the subject, "Do you feel the same or different?" To answer, the subject needs to examine their present experience, and compare it to what it was before, and make their first communication to you a positive one about what they have experienced so far.

If the subject's response is not as described, direct the subject's attention to what they are experiencing in the moment, and encourage a response of some positive effects of the healing that the subject has noticed so far, something that is, in fact, true.

After that, if some degree of symptom remains, the subject can communicate that, and you can again ask the subject to open for the completion of the healing, as they did before, and send White Light to the part of the body that does not yet feel totally right.

Fill that part with White Light, and dissolve the shadows there that have been experienced as discomfort. When that is done, you can again let the subject know that they can open their eyes, and again ask whether they feel the same or different.

This can be continued until the symptom has been totally released, or until a sufficient time has been spent doing this, to make it clear that the healing has so far had all the effects it is likely to have during this healing. See whether other techniques, such as working with chakras or thought forms, are effective in totally releasing the symptoms. Usually, a combination of these techniques can succeed when any one of them alone encounters resistance.

Hold the perception that the positive effects will continue for some time, and that the total effects may, in fact, be shortly manifest. We say that the healing always happens, even when there is resistance to the full immediate release of the symptoms, since the communication and acknowledgment of this resistance can be seen to be a step towards the experience of the full effects of the healing.

When you are using White Light as first aid, the physical position of the subject makes no difference at all, but just the immediate imperative of filling the subject with White Light, to reduce or eliminate the symptom demanding attention. Whenever possible, this can be done while touching the subject anywhere, since the sense of touch does provide a degree of reassurance that is needed and wanted in emergency situations, as well as a vehicle for the feeling of well-being that is provided by the White Light.

If you are not close enough to touch the subject, it is still possible to imagine the subject filled with White Light, creating in yourself the perception that the subject is feeling better and better, and that what had been perceived as a problem is now either totally resolved, or well on the way in that direction, and continuing to improve. As you hold that perception, that thought form of the completed healing goes into the ether, contributing to the co-creation that we call physical external reality, and thus contributing to the actual healing on the physical level. Our perceptions create our reality.

Hold the perception that anything can be healed.

CHAPTER 18

Healing with Chakras and/or Thought Forms

In the classic healing, the healer can use the colors of the chakras to create a model of wellness.

If you see a different color in a chakra from that which is natural for that chakra, you can remove the different color and replace it with the proper color. When each color is in its proper place (Red in the Red Chakra, Orange in the Orange Chakra, etc.), you have created the perception that the subject is experiencing wellness.

(If you have not yet read over the detailed information on the chakras contained in the Appendices, now would be a good time to do so, so you can follow the explanations fully).

When using the colors of the chakras as a model of wellness, you can function in combination with thought forms, or without them. It is all right to function without thought forms, for the idea is that the chakras represent everything happening in the subject's consciousness anyway, so that nothing else is necessary.

Healers who favor working with thought forms and the chakras together claim another level of detail that is available to them concerning what has been happening in the subject's consciousness, and greater responsiveness to the subject's description of symptoms.

When thought forms are used in combination with the chakras, it is still the proper color in each chakra that determines wellness; any thought form that presents itself must be removed, regardless of whether it is seen as good or bad, simply because if it is left there, the final picture is something different from the model of wellness we use.

Sometimes, a thought form will present itself in order for us to communicate something to the subject after the healing, as part of the healing ("There were angels with you in your Indigo Chakra," or "Someone you love was with you in the Green Chakra," for example). When you work with the classic chakra healing as described below, if thought forms present themselves, take care of each one as you encounter it, before moving on to the next chakra.

When the classic form of healing is not practical, as in emergency situations or using healing as first aid, you can most often work with White Light, as described in the previous chapter, or with thought forms, because of the speed and ease with which symptoms can be released with these. Working with thought forms is particularly useful for immediately releasing pain or headaches, for example with pressure valves, while working with chakras gives more detail about the conditions of stress in the specific parts of the subject's consciousness, but takes a bit longer.

While first aid usually involves the use of thought forms, there are times when some chakra work is also used as a first aid. For example, if a subject has left the body (as in the case of an epileptic fit or fainting), you can quickly bring them back into the body by forming the Red Chakra, sending roots into the earth, and bringing the nourishment up into the Red Chakra. Because the Red Chakra is associated with the subject's relationship with the physical body, this usually results in a rapid return.

In the classic chakra healing, begin as you did with the classic **White Light** healing, making certain that the subject is seated with feet flat on the floor, hands open and relaxed on the lap with palms facing up, and eyes closed, reflecting an inner attitude of openness and receptivity.

Begin with the Healing Starting Position, getting the feeling in your hands that tells you that you feel energy, and that a healing can happen. Then, decide that the energy you feel is White Light radiating from your hands.

Place your hands gently on the subject's shoulders, barely making contact, and imagine that you are quickly filling the subject with White Light. During the White Light healing, you did this with the intention of seeing the healing complete when you saw the subject totally filled with White Light, and it probably took between five and fifteen minutes, depending on what you saw and did along the way. Here, the intention is different. You have decided to work with further levels of detail available to you through working with the chakras.

No form of healing is less or more effective than any other. Each can be used to heal anything. Here, filling the subject with White Light gives you the impression that you are entering the consciousness of the subject to its deepest part, and that what you see during the healing will be seen from that deepest part. The filling with White Light may take just one or two minutes, and you may have some picture that tells you that you are at that deepest part, the center of the subject's consciousness. It may be a tube in the center of the subject, or an image of the subject there. As the subject is being filled with White Light, there may, in fact, be some things that are being healed, like armor being released, or a shell opening.

After the subject is filled with White Light, touch the subject in the various parts of the body that correspond to each chakra, not speaking as you work, but rather just seeing what is there, and doing whatever needs to be done to create the perception that the healing has happened. Again, it must be stated that the subject can be healed whether you use touch or not, but here we are describing contact healing, which offers additional levels of communication and reassurance to the subject.

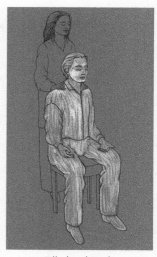

Filled with Light

Because of the sensitivity that so many people have about having their **Red Chakra** touched (it is located at the perineum, between the anus and the sex organs), most healers work more readily at the base of the spine. If there is a serious problem at the level of the Red Chakra, consider touching the subject where they need to be healed, but otherwise, you can work with the base of the spine, or work with your hand under the chair, directly below the area needing to be healed. With your hands in position, imagine a stream of energy coming from your hands or fingers, creating a ball of clear red energy where you know the Red Chakra to be located. If you see another color there, remember what it is, but remove it and replace it with red. Any thought forms are also removed.

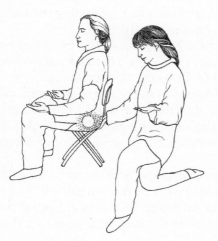

Forming Red Chakra

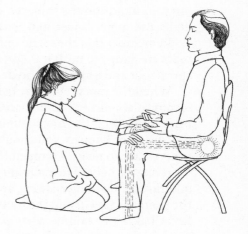

Roots to the Feet

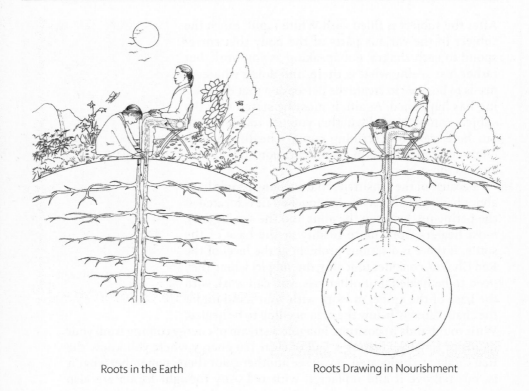

Roots in the Earth   Roots Drawing in Nourishment

When the Red Chakra is in its clear state, ask the Red Chakra to send roots down the subject's legs, to the feet, watching what happens and encouraging the roots if necessary. You can then change your position, placing your hands on the subject's knees, and then feet, imagining the scene under the subject's feet, and changing it if necessary.

Remember that the scene under the subject's feet should be one where roots are happy to be. If it is not, change it until it is. Then, ask the roots to spread out and go deeper and deeper to the source of nourishment.

When the roots touch the ball of energy in the center of the earth, the response should be immediate. The nourishment should immediately begin to flow up the roots and into the subject's legs and Red Chakra. If this does not happen, you should encourage the process, doing whatever is necessary to make it happen.

It may be helpful to maintain an inner dialogue with the subject, asking questions, imagining answers, and talking with the roots in this way. When the energy is flowing up the roots, you can again position your hand at the Red Chakra to examine what is happening there, to assure yourself that the subject is taking in the energy.

For the next few chakras, you can work at either side of the subject, with one hand touching the subject in front, and the other touching the subject from the back. If the back of the chair is in the way, this doesn't matter, since consciousness can move through anything.

At the level of the **Orange Chakra**, imagine a stream of energy coming from each hand, creating a ball of the proper color where you know the Orange Chakra to be. Any thought forms encountered should be taken care of as they present themselves.

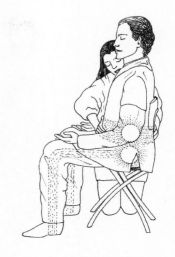

When the Orange Chakra is in its proper state, the procedure is repeated for the **Yellow Chakra**.

Healing the Orange Chakra

Before working on the Green Chakra, and with one hand still touching the Yellow Chakra, place your other hand on the Green Chakra in order to make certain that there is a clear channel between the two chakras, a passage through the membrane mentioned in Chapter 8.

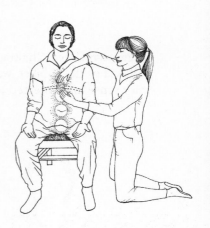

Imagine each chakra as if it is in a room, and ask the ceiling of the Yellow Chakra room to open, as well as the floor of the Green Chakra room. Optimally, the two open, like two iris diaphragms, and the two chakras are able to see each other with just clear space between them. If the subject is defensive, the openings might be locked, and then you must open it with a key. (See diagram: Opening the Passage.)

Any other pictures that do not represent open space between the two chakras must be changed until the energy flows freely between

Opening the Passage

the two. When the membrane is there as a barrier, what the subject experiences, as they move their consciousness between the Yellow Chakra and the Green (between perceptions related to power, control, and freedom to those of love and relating), is resistance in the form of anger, or sadness, or another emotion that can be understood to represent resistance, and which does not feel good. Until the barrier is removed, the membrane of resistance is experienced each time the subject moves their attention between the two chakras.

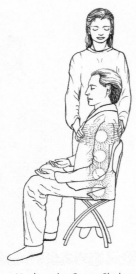

Healing the Green Chakra

When there is a barrier between any two chakras, it represents a barrier in that subject's consciousness between two ideas. Here, it might be a conflict between the ideas of freedom and being in a relationship, or between control and acceptance. Opening the passage makes it easier for the subject to move their attention between the two chakras, and removes the conflict that had existed in their consciousness. The subject then is able to see the compatibility between the two ideas.

After the passage is made between the two chakras, the Green Chakra is healed in the same way as the Orange and Yellow, with one hand touching in front, and one behind, and with energy flowing from both hands, forming a ball of the proper color where they meet. Some healers like to imagine emerald green in their own Green Chakra, sending it down their arms and into the Green Chakra of the subject, watching what happens as they do that. It gives a nice sense of connectedness to both healer and subject.

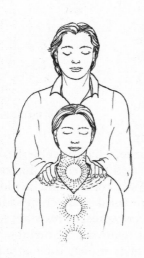

Forming the Blue Chakra

For the **Blue Chakra**, your hands should always be placed on the shoulders, and not in front and behind, so that the subject does not have the sensation of being strangled. With one hand on each shoulder, imagine a stream of energy coming from each hand, forming a ball of sky blue where you know the Blue Chakra to be. You should remove any chains, weights, or any other thought forms as they are encountered.

After the Blue Chakra is as it should be, ask it to put branches down the arms, as you stand to the side of the subject, with one hand at the back of the subject's Blue Chakra, and the other touching the subject's palm on that side. Then, the blue stream of energy should be seen extending beyond the palm, to what appears to be a reasonable distance (to most healers /24–30 feet looks about right).

The procedure is repeated on the other side, and there should be a point at which the two streams of energy meet. If they do not, they must be "aimed" until they do. Sometimes, a scene will appear at the place where the two streams meet, and if so, it represents something that is a goal in the subject's consciousness. It can be important to the subject, and part of their healing, to know what, if anything, you saw there.

For the **Indigo Chakra**, your hands can again be placed in front of and behind the head, at the level of the forehead, and healed in the same way as the Orange, Yellow, and Green.

Some healers like to imagine the Indigo Chakra as a window. They look into the window to see the view inside the room there, and everything in the room should be indigo, midnight blue. If you do this, you should be able to see the subject seated in the center of the room, looking out through the window.

Sometimes, what you see in the room shows the subject's relationship with their house, their vehicle, their physical body, as well as their relationship with spirituality. You should understand what you see there within this context. Remember that the Indigo Chakra represents the subject's view of themselves as the spirit within the body, wearing the biological structure, but being the spirit inside.

The view looking out should show, through an open window, a clear night

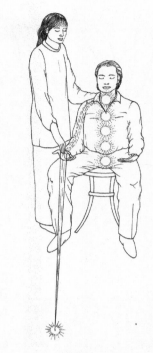

Forming Blue Laser

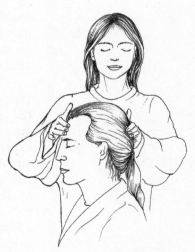

Healing the Indigo Chakra

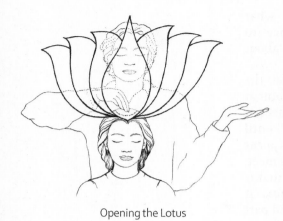

Opening the Lotus

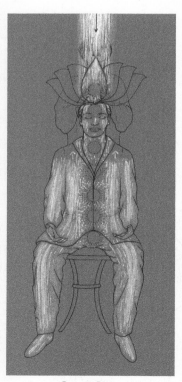

Cosmic Rinse

sky. Any other scene should be changed until it is as it should be. The view looking in through the window shows the subject's self-view in relation to their vehicle, and the view looking out shows the subject's ability to direct their spiritual view outward and apply it to what is happening around them.

With the **Violet Chakra**, one hand is placed at the top of the subject's head, in contact with it, and the violet ball of energy is formed. Afterwards, ask the Violet Chakra to open. Ideally, this happens easily and resembles a lotus opening to its deepest part. If this does not happen, some helmet or barrier needs to be removed, and the request to open repeated.

Finally, with the chakra open as it should be, ask for White Light from above to fill the subject through the Violet Chakra, from the toes up, making each of the chakras, from the red to the violet, glow brighter and clearer than they had before.

When the subject is filled with White Light and overflowing with White Light, and each chakra is glowing bright and clear with the proper color, and no more thought forms are present, you have created the perception that the healing is complete.

Then inform the subject that they can open their eyes when they like, and ask whether they feel the same or different. The subject should be encouraged to notice what is different in their experience of their consciousness and their body, and to make the first communication to you a positive one about what they have experienced so far.

If symptoms remain that have not yet been totally released, you can choose to immediately address these symptoms, or wait until after the subject has received the feedback about what has happened so far.

You can welcome the subject, the new consciousness, into the world with a hug. In this way, the subject has a chance to thank you by placing their heart next to yours, and just feeling the contact, and you have a chance to thank the subject for the opportunity to be the vehicle for the love and energy flowing through you for the subject's healing.

After the feedback is complete, and the symptoms have been released, another hug completes the healing in the consciousness of both you, as the healer, and the subject. When the subject is healed, there is no homework, nothing to work on, no further treatment necessary. They are able to get on with their life. You are able to release any sense of protectiveness or watchfulness over the subject, and can insist on holding the perception that the subject is healed, and no longer requires any further assistance on your part.

In that way, both you and the subject can experience freedom.

Anything can be healed.

CHAPTER 19

Distance Healing

Whatever you are able to do in person with contact healing, you are also able to do at a distance. The degree of distance does not matter, and can be anywhere from some millimeters to thousands of kilometers. After all, you are not working with a physical body, but rather with a consciousness, which has no limitations of time or space.

It is always the consciousness that you see and heal, whether you are working with White Light, chakras, or thought forms. You are working with what the subject is experiencing in their consciousness, and orienting yourself toward returning the subject's consciousness to the experience of wholeness, or wellness. When that happens, the physical body can come into balance with the new configuration of energy created in the healing.

If there are reasons to not touch the subject, such as philosophical or religious reasons, you can function in the same way you would during a contact healing, only keeping your hands from actually touching the body, and working at a distance of some millimeters or centimeters. While you know that physical contact gives you additional levels of communication and has benefits in terms of giving a sense of reassurance to the subject, you must also recognize the times that physical contact can feel intrusive and a violation of the subject's boundaries. Then, you must decide that the healing that is done in another way will have maximum effectiveness as well, and that you will have all the tools and dimensions you need to work with, in order to create the perfect healing. Then, it is so.

Even when working at a distance of some millimeters or centimeters, with the subject physically present in the chair, you will see all that you would see just as if you were touching the subject, but you will just have a different sense of contact.

Since you are working with the consciousness, rather than the physical body, you are able to do the same thing when the subject is not physically located in the chair. You can work with a physically empty chair, imagining the subject seated there, and you will see and feel everything the same as if the subject were seated there, with you working at a distance of some centimeters, not actually touching the subject.

You would still begin with the Healing Starting Position, feeling the energy in your hands, deciding that it's White Light, resting your hands above where the subject's shoulders would be, and imagining filling the subject with White Light.

You would still see the same pictures in the subject's consciousness, because it is still the consciousness with which you are working. To optimize the interaction, you can let the subject know when the healing is to take place, so the subject can consciously leave themselves open at that time to receive the healing.

If the subject does not do that, the healing still takes place at the level of the ether, until they are open to receive the beneficial effects, usually when they have gone to sleep, and the effects of the healing can manifest at that time. Naturally, it is always useful and helpful to offer the subject the feedback about what you saw, what you did, and what it means to you, so that they can orient themselves more easily to the new consciousness in which they experience their wholeness.

In the same way as working with White Light at a distance, you can work with thought forms and chakras, imagining that the subject is seated in the physically empty chair in front of you. At first, it may feel a bit bizarre to work in this way, but as soon as you feel the energy moving, experience seeing the energy system of the subject, and validate the feedback that you have seen, you will know

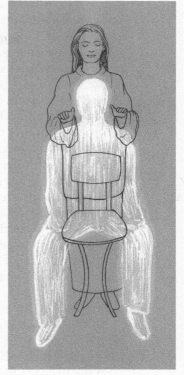

Distance Healing

that your effectiveness is not diminished by any distance. You will know that in the same way, you can heal anyone in the world, wherever they are, at any time.

Some healers find it more comfortable, however, to work on the distant consciousness with the help of a surrogate subject in the chair. That is, someone agrees to sit in the chair to take the place of the actual subject who is being healed, and then the energy system of the actual subject is seen, rather than the energy system of the surrogate subject. Then, the surrogate subject, even if they do not know what needed to be healed in the actual subject, can give you feedback about what they experienced during the healing.

The surrogate subject may have felt things in their body related to the symptoms being healed, or seen images that you will be able to relate to, in terms of what was healed in the distant subject. While this is usually done quite consciously, by asking someone to serve as a surrogate subject, it may sometimes happen spontaneously, and without your knowledge. You may suddenly recognize that the energy system you have seen and have been working with is not at all related to the intended subject, the person in the chair. All that was seen was correct, even though the person in the chair did not relate at all to the feedback. It is as though the person in the chair had agreed to be there for the healing of someone else, although the person in the chair may have received benefits as well.

It might even be the consciousness of someone in the person's life, such as a parent or other relative, who needed a healing, and about whom the person had been anxious. Then, one of the effects of the distance healing that happened through the person in the chair, was the release of their own anxiety. Healing has many forms.

Since all of the healings described so far involve a sense of connectedness between healer and subject, we can say that other forms of healing are also possible, given the same sense of connectedness. Thus through hearing a subject's voice on the telephone, you can form a connection with their consciousness and a healing can happen that way. You still can imagine working with White Light, chakras, and thought forms, at the same time, feeling the subject's consciousness as you work, and receiving immediate feedback about the effectiveness of what you are doing.

Of course, working with someone's photo can trigger the same sense of connectedness if the subject is someone that you know or have met previously, and the healing can then happen in that way.

If the distance healing involves a subject with whom you have had no experience of contact, a photo can be used to "find" the subject's consciousness, and the healing can happen. In fact, if all you are given is the subject's name and some information about them, that can be all that is necessary to locate the subject's consciousness and perform the healing. The information can be about the subject's symptom, or age, or some physical attributes.

Then it's as if you are asking Universal Consciousness to find a being with that name and information, and Universal Consciousness returns the "address" of the subject. Then, you can ask the person who provided the name of the subject about other attributes of the subject, to make certain you have the right one. Example: "Does this person have red hair? Yes? Okay, now we can begin."

Some healers who have achieved a certain level of evolution and therefore have a pretty good sense of who they are use yet another kind of distance healing. This is empathic healing, and knowing who you are and what is true for you is a necessary prerequisite. In this type of healing, you feel connected to the subject with a sense of empathy, feeling the subject's experience as if it were your own. It's as if you are in the body and consciousness of the subject, experiencing what the subject is experiencing. Naturally, to know that the consciousness you are experiencing is not your own, you must know your own consciousness well enough to know that what is being experienced has no relation to tensions in your own consciousness. If you know that the experience you feel is not yours, you can ask whose it is, and then recognize whose consciousness you are wearing. You may notice yourself walking or standing the way you know the subject does, or you may recognize the subject's face in your own face.

You then know that when you are connected like that to the subject, when the subject experiences the release of the symptom, you will feel the release within your own experience as well.

In the same way, you can decide that when you release the tension from your own consciousness, and the connection is there with the subject, the subject will experience the same release at the same time.

Obviously, the door is open to other forms of distance healing, such as healing with a look, when the look on the part of the healer is one which chooses to see the subject as whole and insists on holding that perception, or healing with just a thought, in the same way.

As you work more and more in these realms of healing, it will become more and more evident to you that there is no limit to the ways in which you can use your own perceptions to bring another to the experience of wholeness. You will also realize that when you are able to affect biological structure with your thoughts, you will be able to use your consciousness to change anything at all in the physical world. Other dimensions of healing will become apparent. You will be able to see situations that present themselves to you for healing, and you will be able to see the form of healing required for that situation, and use it.

And, you will be able to do it from no matter where in the world you happen to be.

With sufficient practice, to establish a sense of trust in your subjective impressions (the tools that you work with in healing), you will feel as comfortable working with distance healing, as with the most simple contact healing.

Anything can be healed.
You can heal anything.

CHAPTER 20

Self-Healing

Anything you are able to do for another, you are able to do for yourself. After all, you are the same kind of energy system as the others you have been successful at healing. All is possible when you are able to see your own body in the same way you see the bodies of others, as just the vehicle for the consciousness within, and furthermore, just part of an energy system.

Ideally, of course, you will never need healing, if you stay in touch with yourself, always being yourself, understanding your consciousness and the language it uses, and always responding consciously. While it is true that not so many beings on the earth have so far achieved this level of perfection and optimal functioning, it is also true that there is no reason to believe that it is anything but available to you in any moment, including this one, now.

If some symptom does present itself to you, you can have some compassion for yourself, recognizing that you are still learning, and have not yet finished working on yourself. If you see that the symptom to be healed in you is a repeat of something that happened before, you will know that you need to change something in your consciousness, so that the same thing does not happen again. You will also know what it is that needs to change.

You can allow yourself to be reminded many times, just to be certain, or you can choose to get the message earlier and earlier, staying in touch with your inner directional system, your intuition.

You can either choose to allow yourself to be healed by another, or to do the healing yourself. Do whatever is necessary to release yourself from the symptom, and return yourself to the state of being in which you are happy and healthy. It's your natural state.

The healing can be in the form of first aid, or in the form of a healing meditation.

When healing yourself as a form of first aid, you will be able to remove headaches and pains in the same way that you would if you were working with another subject. You can use thought forms, pressure valves, and so on. You must choose to see yourself in that moment as only an energy system, and not be emotionally involved in the symptom you are releasing. Then, you can just lift away the ache or pain, and feel it go. You can heal cuts or bruises by holding the area, and imagining the healing taking place, watching the process as blood vessels reseal, as flesh mends, insisting then on seeing it as healed, and deciding that it is so.

If it is a headache that you are releasing, and you feel it leave your consciousness, you will notice that certain thoughts leave your consciousness at the same time. It will be like a cloud leaving. You will know that they were the thoughts associated with the symptom, which had created it. Do not chase the thoughts, wanting to remember what they had been. Just watch them go, and experience the clearer consciousness that remains.

If you are spending time with one foot in each reality, sometimes being in one bubble and sometimes another, you will be able to see the effects of your thoughts. You will see that when you have that particular thought, you will experience that particular symptom. When you release the symptom, you will feel the thought that created it leaving, also, being replaced by another perception that is clearer for you. You will then be able to keep your attention on the ideas and consciousness you experience when you are symptom-free, and maintain that as your usual state of consciousness, who you really are, and what is real and true for you.

If there is some emotional involvement with the symptom, because it is happening within your body, the effects of the healing may take a bit longer to manifest, but it will still be much more rapid than leaving the symptom to be handled only in physical cause-and-effect reality.

When you choose to heal yourself using meditation as the form of healing, it will not interfere with any medical treatment you are receiving, but rather will accelerate the process. You can use, for example, the Chakra Meditation found in Section V of this book. When you do, realize that the chakras are only representing portions of your consciousness, and that therefore any change you bring about in the chakras must be accompanied by a corresponding change in the consciousness you experience as your own.

When you know that you have a symptom, you know that there is a part of your consciousness that is not clear. Therefore, when you look at the chakra representing that part of your consciousness, you must be able to see the non-clarity represented in some way, as a thought form or as some color different from that which is "natural" for that chakra. If you experience some physical symptom, but the chakra seems to be perfect when you look at it, you must know that you are not seeing what is really there, and you must adjust your perceptions to acknowledge what is true for you.

When you do see what is there, you can change it, and the effect can be experienced immediately. Thus, it is as possible to release any symptom within yourself with the same rapidity as when you are healing someone else by working on chakras. Of course, this requires a willingness on your part to release the aspects of consciousness that created the symptom, in favor of the experience of yourself that reflects harmony and balance.

It also requires a willingness to look at the situation that created the symptom in the first place, and see it in a new way. In that way, you accept the healing, and you know what needs to be different from now on.

If you are more comfortable with gradual change, the meditation has the effect of establishing a model of wholeness through putting into the chakras the colors natural to them, and each time that is done, allowing yourself to accept the changes to some degree. Then each time the meditation is done, the colors that are there at the beginning of the meditation are closer and closer to what they should be. This continues until you are experiencing your wholeness, and seeing the colors that are "natural" to the chakras throughout the meditation.

The idea is to approach the meditation with the intention of being present throughout the process. If you notice, however, that during certain parts of the meditation, you experience thoughts that have a tendency to distract you, you will know that you need to redirect your attention to completing your intention, which is, being present with what you are there to do, and what you have decided to do.

Gradually, you can notice less and less of a tendency to allow yourself to be distracted, and you then know that you are more in control of your own consciousness. You can also know that you are clearer with the parts of your consciousness that the chakra represents, where you had allowed yourself to be distracted before. Eventually, you are able to be totally present with what you are there to do, with your highest priority—i.e. your healing—and you can also experience the aspects of your healing that this success creates.

It helps if you set a time frame as a goal. This can be any reasonable amount of time—week or a month, for example. You can decide that at the end of that time, you will see where you are, and measure the degree of healing that has taken place. You have decided that there will be improvement, and the only question remaining is the degree. Then, you can have a sense of when the process will be complete.

In the experience of this writer, the time I decided for my healing was two months, to release totally a tumor that had been growing in my spinal cord, at the level of my neck, and so the degree of improvement was geared to the time available for its completion. Finally, after two months, it was necessary to decide that the process was now complete, and to receive the feedback from the medical authorities that had diagnosed the tumor, that it was no longer there. It was obviously also necessary to deeply promise to myself to make whatever changes in my life that were necessary for the release of the symptoms, and to keep that promise.

The same is true of any person healing any symptom, even though the severity may be less.

Apply the same principles to yourself that are discussed in the various chapters of this book describing the healing process as a co-creation, knowing while you do that you are playing the part of both the healer and the subject. And watch the healing happen.

You know that anything can be healed.

Other Dimensions

CHAPTER 21

Mirroring
(Politics of Communication)

When you offer feedback after the healing to the subject, certain dynamics of communication become evident. You know that you must not impose your view on the subject, but just offer the view from your own bubble. The subject may agree that your view expresses what they have felt or they may say they have not experienced what you have described to them.

If your view is one the subject can relate to, the communication can be accepted as a valid communication. That is, what you as the healer experienced and communicated was also reflected in the subject's experience. The subject could relate to what had been described. In addition, the receiver of the communication was as interested in hearing what was said as the transmitter of the information was in offering it.

If the subject does not relate to what was communicated, or has no experience of it, it is useful that they say so. In this case, your experience as the healer in what was communicated was not reflected in the experience of the subject. Still, the receiver of the information was as interested in hearing what was said as the transmitter of the information was in offering it. The communication was still accepted. We also know that perhaps some time afterward, the subject might realize that what was communicated does, in fact, relate to them, although it might be in a way different from what you as the healer had expressed.

You must remember that you were expressing the view as seen through and colored by your own bubble. The information given in the feedback, though, must make sense to the one who was healed. The picture may be the same, but have a different interpretation.

When the subject does not relate to what you have communicated, you must examine the nature of your own perceptions. Perhaps the subject will recognize something later on, but then again, maybe not. We know that we are each in a bubble, the filter of our perceptions, and that the inside of our bubble is a mirror.

Could you have been seeing a reflection of yourself? Could what you described in the communication relate to you? Could you recognize it as a biased point of view, or one based on your past perceptions or prejudices?

Perhaps, and perhaps not, but it is important that you ask yourself the questions.

If you repeatedly communicate the same sort of information during different healings, you must take a close look at the degree to which the information relates to you, and whether you need to take some advice from yourself, applying in your own life the advice and feedback you have been communicating to others during their healings.

Even when the subject has accepted as their own all of the information you communicated, you can still choose to notice any consistent themes, and ask yourself anyway whether the communication relates to you as well, or whether it can possibly be relevant to you. You can use the healing of the subject to give yourself feedback about how to handle the issues in your own life. It can look to you as though the subject has had the same problems, but has perhaps gone further into stress with them, experiencing the effects of that stress, perhaps even as deadly symptoms.

You can then see where you, yourself, might be heading if you do not change direction, and find resolution for yourself. You can see the subject with compassion, and speak with the subject as you would to yourself, knowing that the subject has helped you with your own healing. You can also sincerely thank the subject afterward for the experience of the healing.

Even when the similarities between the subject's symptoms and your life are not apparent in the moment of experience, you may notice that you have been attracting a particular type of healing. Has there been something that all of these healings have had in common? Has it been different from the types of healings that other healers have attracted?

If you notice some common theme, you can pay attention to that. If the feedback from those other healings is not remembered, you can pay attention to the healings you will attract to yourself after that, and know that the Universe is providing you with everything you need to heal your own life while healing others.

We can say that we attract to ourselves others who bring out from us information we need to hear for ourselves. Thus, the source of all we need to know is in our own consciousness. Our perceptions are all that we need to give us all the information we need about how to conduct our own lives. In that way, we are each our own guru, our own master, and our own guide. All that has been needed was to know how to decode and understand what our own perceptions have been showing us. Seeing things in this way, we can experience a sense of real freedom, while taking full responsibility for ourselves.

You may offer your services to those who appear to need it, while at the same time leaving the others the right to accept or reject your offer of help.

If the others choose to not accept the help, you can examine your own perceptions of the others for possible adjustment, and for what these perceptions show you.

For example, you may have the idea that someone needs a healing because their values differ from yours. Perhaps the person is angry in that moment, but feeling okay about that, or perhaps their way of dealing with money, sexuality or relationships is different from yours.

You might decide that this person is not clear in their consciousness, but they might not feel the same way. If they are not interested in accepting a healing, or do not share your perception that a healing is needed, you must consider that perhaps your own prejudices need to be healed.

If it's clear that the other person is experiencing the effects of a physical symptom, and therefore obviously needs a healing but does not want one for some reason, you can choose to see them with compassion, and not press your offer. Perhaps their healing needs to happen another time, or another way, or with another healer.

It's interesting to apply the same dynamics of communication to everyday life. After all, isn't it still about each of the participants in an event expressing their own experience, and what is true for them? When the mutual respect of the healing transaction is applied to interpersonal communication, we recognize a similarity of dynamics.

When there is communication, it is supposed that both parties are interested in the communication. When your perceptions of another evokes in you a desire to tell something to them, ask yourself whether they are as eager to hear the advice as you are to give it. If so, there is a potential for communication. When the person who is intended to receive the communication is less interested in hearing it than you are in communicating it, you have something to examine. Apparently, the words want to come out, but they do not want to be heard by the other.

Who, then, are the words for? Perhaps yourself. Maybe later on, the other can ask for the feedback. Then you can complete the communication, and each of you can consider the degree to which the information communicated relates to you. When you are directing words towards others, you can notice when you are talking to yourself. Then you can listen as well, knowing that you're about to give yourself some excellent advice that will help you with something that has been a problem. You can even thank the other person for having evoked this advice from you to yourself.

If you are the intended receiver of the information, you can remember that everyone is entitled to their own opinion, and an opinion is all that is being communicated. The other person is just expressing their point of view. If the communication arouses resistance, perhaps something about the resistance needs to be examined.

You can always ask yourself whether what was communicated relates to you, or whether it is apparent that the one making the communication is looking into the magic mirror, and talking to themselves.

If a decision is made to communicate, and to do so clearly, the receiver can choose to hear what was said, and if their own experience is something different from what was communicated, they can say so.

When both participants in a communication feel free to express their own view and their experience of what was communicated by the other, misunderstandings can be cleared up, and disagreements based on these misunderstandings can be resolved. Each one can understand the other's bubble. When each of the positions is acknowledged, another level of communication is possible.

Using these same principles, we can examine the nature of our own perceptions, and learn from them, even when we have not externalized these perceptions in a verbal communication with another being.

The filter of our perceptions surrounds us, like a bubble, as you know quite well by now. Everything we experience is perceived through this filter. This filter colors everything we perceive. We can say that at least some of the time, we do not see things as they are, but rather as we are. We project onto others our perceptions of their motivations, and what we believe is good for them to do or not do.

When we feel resistance to someone, we can ask ourselves what the characteristics are of that person. What kind of person are they? What words could be used to describe them? Then, we can ask ourselves whether those words could be used to describe us, and we might feel a bit embarrassed to discover that, in fact, we remember situations where those words would have certainly described us.

We might say to ourselves that our motivations were proper at that time, and we did what we did for a good reason. Then, we must also consider that the other person is probably justifying their actions in the same way, and perhaps having the same motivations.

We are then able to see the other as a reflection of ourselves, and when we do that, much (if not all) of the resistance disappears. Where there had been a wall, a barrier to communication, there is now a doorway, a possibility of communication. We are able to see the other with compassion, and we can accept the wisdom that comes with this compassion. We have been able to raise our perceptions from the level of the solar plexus, and perceptions of judgement, power, and control, to the level of the heart, and perceptions of compassion and relating. We are more easily able to see the other with acceptance. Resistance disappears.

We had thought, perhaps, that we knew what the other should do differently. However, with the exception of actions that threaten the social organism in which we function, all we must really concern ourselves with as free beings is our own actions and attitudes. In accepting others as they are, we are still free to decide for ourselves our own proper course of action—what we should do.

If you relate to the process described here, it is easy to see that you had been putting yourself in the other's place, and saying, "If I were that other person, I should be doing something different from that." According to the values with which you live, if you were that other person, you would be doing something wrong. What you may not have considered is that the other person may be living with other values, and that what they have been doing might be working for them, according to their own values. That person brought out from you advice that would be good for you to follow. We can say, then, that you were talking to yourself. Were you listening, too?

The world is full of people who are walking around talking to themselves, but only some of them are listening. When we realize this, we continue to walk around talking to ourselves, but now we also listen.

While this mirroring aspect to our perceptions is generally buried below the level of awareness for most people, at the usual levels of perception of the first three chakras, it does become a direct experience from the level of the Green Chakra, the chakra of the heart, and its aspect of relating. We directly perceive others as reflections of ourselves, and all of the processes described here become directly evident.

We are able to see ourselves in the other's place, and speak to them as if speaking to ourselves. We can experience more compassion in our perceptions of the other, with the realizations triggered by that compassion, and the wisdom that it generates. We are then able to communicate more freely, and more easily, and use this communication as a vehicle for true relating. Then, we are able to love more.

Love heals.

Anything can be healed.

CHAPTER 22

Winds and Waves—Creation and Co-creation

Everything begins with consciousness. Your consciousness. From your point of view as an individual, then, everything that happens in your life, and everything that happens in your body, begins with something happening in your own consciousness.

If you look behind you in your life, at the things that have happened, you can recognize that somewhere, these events have reflected deep decisions you had already made. Reality manifested to carry out those decisions. It's as if you have been walking through a dream, which has been responding to your deep desires and choices. In your dream, yours is the only consciousness involved, and everything around you is just a projection of that consciousness. The other characters in your dream, also, are just projections of your consciousness, acting out their parts in response to what you have decided, or to what you believe to be true.

As the consciousness creating the dream, the projector creating the movie, you are the creator, agreeing to play the parts of the director, the actor, and the audience, all at the same time. Everything you decide will be acted out and played by you, and you can even review your own movie, and decide how good it is, and whether it is just perfect the way it is, or if it would be even better rewritten in some way. From this point of view, as seen from your Violet Chakra, your crown chakra, the single point of consciousness experiencing "I am," the dreamer dreaming the dream—you are all there is.

From another point of view, we can say that just as you are a consciousness projecting your dream around yourself, your bubble, your sphere of experience, the other characters in your movie are doing the same thing. Each of them is a consciousness projecting their bubble around themselves, and somehow, interacting with others doing the same thing, in a marvelous and intricate, perfectly functioning, well-oiled organic machine.

The bubbles interpenetrate each other, and where they meet, where the scripts overlap, and the scenery, they create a three-dimensional hologram we agree to call physical external reality. Then, the events that happen in this external reality are the result of the decisions made by each of the consciousnesses involved in those events. We need to acknowledge not only ourselves as creators, but each and every other consciousness as well, in the same way. Seeing all beings as co-creators is a view from the Indigo Chakra.

This acknowledgment of self and others as creators is necessary for spiritual evolution. In doing this, you will have the means to explore particular parts of your own consciousness not otherwise accessible. How, for example, would you be able to explore communication if there were no other being but yourself?

By exploring co-creation, you can get beyond your own subjective view, and benefit from the wisdom of a larger view, that of the group consciousness concerned with the well-being of all its members, the view of the organism protecting all of its parts.

When watching the events in physical reality, the things having a tendency to happen or to not happen around you, you can learn much by personifying these energies, that is, characterizing them as if you were interacting with another consciousness. This other consciousness can be an individual, or your Spirit, or any group consciousness such as the spirit of a country or of a city, you choose to examine in this way.

Then, you can ask yourself what seems to be the nature of the interaction. Does it seem that this group consciousness is pleased with your interaction, encouraging it, or is it communicating another message?

What is the nature of this view from the Indigo Chakra? When we consider only your consciousness as a creator of infinite ability, we can say that when you make a decision or set a goal, the fulfillment of that goal exists somewhere. You have created it with your intention, and with the picture of fulfillment that you have placed in your consciousness you have begun to move towards that fulfillment.

We can also say that events in the dream, the movie around you, seem to be responding to your intention, so that these outer events, too, are moving you to the completion of your goals, set in motion by the decisions in your consciousness, like winds and waves on the ocean of co-created reality. You decide things—and they happen:

Decision "A" —> Manifestation "A"

What happens, then, when two creators (each of infinite ability) have made different decisions? Reality will, of course, have a tendency to flow toward the completion of the intentions of both creators.

The two different intentions might be complementary or opposing. If they are complementary, each of the creators is strengthening and reinforcing the other, and what they have each decided will have more of a tendency to happen. The winds and waves will be stronger.

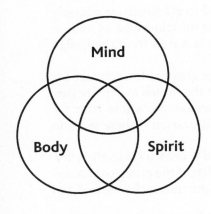

In a healing, for example, the manifestation of the agreement of intentions results in the release of symptoms, and much faster than would have happened as the result of the decisions of only one of the consciousnesses, with its limited view.

When the intentions are not aligned, things happen in a different way. The non-alignment can be the result of either conscious decisions, or of feelings and reactions. Remember, we are each a single consciousness, but at the same time, we are also each described as mind, body, and spirit combined:

- The body represents physical cause-and-effect reality, the degree to which we place our faith in what happens according to the laws of chemistry, biology, and physics.
- The mind represents our basic beliefs, our ideas, which can be used to limit ourselves—or to overcome the limits imposed by physical reality.
- The spirit can be used to represent not only the spirit and spiritual realities, but also the emotions and our emotional responses to events.

As we have explained, reality manifests according to your goals, because of the pictures you have put into your consciousness. It can also manifest according to your fears. We can say that holding a picture in your consciousness of what you are afraid of will give it more of a tendency to happen because you are energizing that picture, putting attention on it, and being glued to that picture with your fears.

You can use the realization that the glue, the fear, is attracting that which you fear, making it more likely to manifest, to motivate yourself to release the fear, and to hold instead a picture of a different event or a more favorable outcome.

Instead of holding a picture of your lover leaving, for example, you can insist on holding the picture of your lover staying and being happy with you, energizing that as a manifestation, and if it is done in a way that satisfies your lover's needs as well, they will have a tendency to agree to your picture.

In considering co-creation involving equals, we must remember that it takes two to say yes and only one to say no. Co-creation is a reality by agreement, a paradigm of mutual consent.

In terms of healing, when we are considering it as a manifestation of two creators, if the subject is afraid to let go of old ideas, the mere fact that they are holding on to them can diminish your effectiveness as the healer, and the healing will have less of a tendency to happen. We can say that there will be resistance to the healing happening. Of course, if you have some limiting ideas of what you are able to do, there will be the same result, that is, resistance to the healing happening.

This can manifest as a tendency for the symptoms to not release, or to release more slowly, or it can manifest as a tendency for the healing to not happen. That is, a tendency for the healer to not complete the job, or for external events to flow in the direction of encouraging the healing to not happen.

Loud noises during the healing, for example, that might have a tendency to distract the attention of the participants, and thus interrupt the healing, could be seen as an example of resistance in the consciousness of at least one of the participants. It would manifest in the physical universe as a tendency for the healing to not happen.

Another possible form of resistance could be for you to get dizzy, feeling unable to continue with the healing. During the healing, when you have aligned your intention with that of the subject to see the subject healed, and have no personal purpose other than that, everything that happens in the physical universe during the healing is the manifestation of the consciousness of the subject. The subject is, in that activity, the center of the universe, and it is their consciousness that is creating the movie. We would therefore say that it was the consciousness of the subject creating the loud noises, and even the dizziness of the healer, as distractions.

As you remove the resistance from the consciousness of the subject, manifestation in the physical universe comes into balance with that, and changes in favor of encouraging the healing process. The loud noises stop. You no longer feel dizzy. Things tend to flow again.

Of course, we can also say that everything that happens during the healing is the result of the consciousness of the healer, who is ultimately responsible for it all, and it is a valid point of view. It does not, however, answer the question of why a healer working on two healings of similar symptoms, one after the other, will experience more ease with one of the healings than the other. If we can say that the healer brings the same ingredients to each healing, we must conclude that the difference in results is the effect of what was happening in the consciousness of the subject.

If resistance arises during the healing, it is for both participants in the healing to decide to affirm to themselves their desire to complete the healing and to remove the resistance. The subject does this by choosing to open more, and you as the healer do this by reaffirming your intention to see this being healed, suspending limiting ideas, and redirecting your attention, when necessary, to completing your intended activity, which is the healing.

The co-creation of the healing is also an example of how the same principles apply to other aspects of your experience. What is the explanation, for example, when those things you have decided in your life have had a tendency to find completion in a way different than you had envisioned? Sometimes it can be better than you thought, and sometimes not really as good. When it is better than you thought, it can be apparent that there was another consciousness involved, a benevolent one, helping you. You can decide that this other consciousness was God, or your spirit, or Fate.

You can also ask yourself who would be happy to see these results besides you, and decide that the winds and waves set in motion by their consciousness were reinforcing yours. Everybody won. You got by with a little help from your friends.

What happens, though, when Decision A results in Manifestation B, which is less than what you decided? Would this be the result of God, or your spirit? These entities, clearly, are working on your behalf. Everything directed by Spirit is for your benefit, whether or not you notice the benefit at the time. You could choose to find the benefit, and the justification for this set of events, or decide that it will be discovered later in time, when the full effects of the event are known.

If the manifestation was less than what represented success to you, you could first look inside yourself, seeing whether there were any limiting beliefs or inhibiting ideas which would explain the events. Were you holding yourself back somewhere? After all, God helps those that help themselves. Limiting ideas can always be changed in favor of others that encourage success, and then it is possible to look forward to a different manifestation in the future.

If we choose to see the Universe manifesting as a group consciousness, a co-creation, it is interesting to notice who would have been happy to see that things happened as they did, either from their conscious intentions or from their emotional reactions.

We could say that the things happening in the other consciousness were creating winds and waves interfering with yours, creating more complex vectors and forces that had a tendency to move things in another direction than that intended by you. After all, the other is a creator also.

To own your own power, we would also have to say that you had allowed yourself to be influenced or affected by the consciousness of someone else whose interests were not in accord with yours, someone who wanted something different to happen than what you really wanted. You would then have the choice of making yourself transparent to these forces or disengaging yourself from the other consciousness, or negotiating with the other consciousness to resolve the apparently different intentions into a solution that worked well for both. Otherwise, it would just be a test of power, and of who could maintain their own certainty or create doubt in the other, weakening them. Certainty enhances manifestation.

Negotiating could result in the setting of new goals that better serve the purposes of both consciousnesses, and therefore have the effect of aligning intentions in a win–win situation, as in a healing, which both could feel good about agreeing to.

That would be like being a wind-surfer riding the winds and waves, so that no matter in which direction they are moving they bring you to whatever destination you choose. Riding the winds and waves, surfing, requires that you be totally present in the moment of experience, conscious and vigilant, aware of not only what is happening inside you, but also what is happening in the manifestation of reality around you. This is a view from the Blue Chakra, the first level of perception at which one notices an interaction with another level of intelligence.

When the circumstances of that moment seem to most encourage a response from you, it is as though the entire movie has stopped, and the next decision you make will decide all events that follow. It is as though you had gone into the ocean with your surfboard, and the wave has come, the optimal moment to act, the cusp, and you must decide in that moment whether to ride the wave, or wait for the next one.

The moment does not last forever. If you decide to wait, or to not decide, the wave continues on its way, and you must wait for another optimal moment, if there is one. Sometimes the wave was one of a kind, the chance of a lifetime. Perhaps if you have faith and patience, there can be another wave, even better, another cusp, and if and when it comes, there will be another perfect moment or time to act.

When the wave comes, you can have an idea of its size by recognizing the possibilities of where it is going, according to goals you had set and decisions you had made, and how this is the answer to these goals and decisions. The quality of the ride will then depend upon your skill in remaining present, responding to conditions in the immediate moment of experience, and choosing to keep moving with those things that have a tendency to happen in that direction.

The healer and the subject are creating the winds and the waves, and the moment of coming together for the healing is creating the opportunity for the decision to ride this wave. It's a short ride that might last only a few minutes, but it's an exciting one, and it does have its far-reaching effects, changing someone's life forever, and perhaps even both lives, in a positive direction.

It's a positive rush. Go for it.

Anything can be healed.

CHAPTER 23

Healing as a Meditation

Meditation is an exercise in inner discipline during which you focus your consciousness, your attention, in a particular way to achieve a particular beneficial effect.

Some people might meditate to achieve a quieter mind or to use their consciousness as a tool to achieve a goal. Some use it to restore harmony to the body, to know the different spiritual dimensions of their own being, to know God, to experience God Consciousness, to achieve Illumination, to know and experience transcendent love or realization, or to understand the nature of physical reality. Some use it to achieve mastery of their consciousness by being able to maintain attention on a single thing, whether it's a word, an idea, a symbol, or their breath—or nothing at all. Of course, there are more reasons than this, but you get the idea.

You begin the experience by emptying yourself of all personal considerations and all personal purposes, deciding to be totally present in the experience, living the function of the healer, being there totally for the subject. What the healer wants for the subject is a reflection of what the subject wants for themselves.

While the motives may sound noble, we are not speaking here of morals or ethics, but only the primary motivating force, the main reason for taking part in the activity. The healing is done for its own sake, and while there may be certain benefits afterwards for you as the healer (you have pride in what you were able to achieve, or you have realized something about your own consciousness, or have gone beyond your own self-imposed limits, or you are paid as a form of exchange, etc.), consideration of these benefits must be secondary to the main purpose, which is about being there to see the subject healed, and choosing to participate in the process in order to see that achieved.

In the first interaction between you and the subject, there is a coming together of two beings of infinite ability, and while you have certain skills the other may not yet have learned, the other is no less a creator. The subject's consciousness has affected their own biological structure in some way, putting it out of balance, and you are going to use your consciousness to have a different effect on it, repairing the damage that had been created. The interaction should reflect the mutual respect due to both beings.

By choosing to enter the experience of the healing, you set an intention, a goal, and must maintain attention on and movement towards that goal, even when there are distracting influences, whether they be external events (noise, for example), self-doubt, or distracting thoughts about the subject (they are ugly, or sexy, or strange).

Any thoughts taking your attention away from what you are doing must be recognized as distractions and released, and attention redirected to the activity at hand—healing the subject. You should, however, acknowledge and not resist persistent distractions, so that you can consider what the message is in terms of the healing that is happening. When these distractions are acknowledged, they usually disappear, and even in those rare moments when they do not, they cease to be distractions. They are then just there as background.

When your thoughts are about things seeming to have nothing to do with the healing (last night's television program, or yesterday's argument, or tomorrow's rent), you can consider what that has to do with the person's healing. Perhaps the thought about that television program, for example, was dropped into your consciousness because it has something to do with the part of the subject's energy system being healed in that moment.

As an empathic experience, the thoughts in your consciousness can be parallel to what is happening in the consciousness of the subject, set in motion by them as a tuning fork sets in motion another which is at the same frequency, in the experience we know as empathy. It is important that you express all your impressions. The dynamics of the feedback will give the subject the opportunity to express whether that relates to them or not.

Characteristics of the subject that might be judged as something bad, you must insist on seeing as just something that has not yet been healed. By removing judgments and expectations from your own consciousness, you are left with perceptions of acceptance.

Acceptance is love. Love heals.

In this atmosphere of acceptance, you are able to freely enter the subject's consciousness, and they can feel comfortable about allowing this to happen, because they do not feel the resistance and separation caused by the judgments and expectations. They feel only your sincere desire to help them. They feel your consciousness to the degree that you are in theirs.

The two consciousnesses are, after all, together in this experience, one inside the other, each open to the other. During the healing, you are open to all impressions that present themselves. For example, even though you might expect to see certain things, you know that seeing what is there is more important than seeing only what you thought would be there. Even though you may have decided, during the discussion of the symptoms to be healed, which chakras are probably involved in that symptom, and what you might see during the healing, there may be surprises. Experience, not ideas, shows us what is real for us.

After the healing, you see what results you have achieved. When the results are remarkable, even according to your standards, you can ask yourself what you did right that resulted in that particular quality of results. Perhaps it was about being more present, perhaps trusting the Universe, going beyond self-imposed limits, or opening to let the love flow. Your perceptions will show you what your success was due to, and what you can do in future healings to assure a comparable level of success.

If you believe in God, you can point to the healing as evidence of what is possible with that. If you have a different philosophical structure, you can use the healing as evidence of what you are personally capable of, after limiting ideas are removed, and, therefore, evidence of what we are all capable of.

Any observers to the healing may have noticed different reasons for the success of the healer from those you noticed. They will have noticed what they could do to achieve the same level of success, seen through the filter of their bubble.

You can ask yourself what would happen if you moved through an entire day in the way you moved through this successful healing, doing the same thing that you know was successful, creating remarkable effects, while enjoying a very particular state of consciousness. You can also ask yourself how you enjoyed that state of consciousness during the healing, compared to what you have experienced as your "normal" way of being.

For a while, you may have two states of consciousness to which you can relate, your "healing" consciousness, and your "normal" consciousness, and you will be able to see the two side by side. If the "healing" consciousness feels better, and shows you a better quality of life, one that feels better and is filled with remarkable experiences benefitting you as well as others, it will be only a matter of time before your orientation will reflect more and more of what feels better to you.

Moving through a day as you would move through a healing might be for only one or two days a week at first, if those are the days you function as a healer, and then perhaps on other days when no "formal" healings have been scheduled just for the experience of knowing what a day looks like from that point of view.

On days when you may not be feeling in top form, and the Universe offers you a healing in which to participate, you can notice how much better you feel when you put your own stuff "on the shelf" by just being there for the healing. You may also notice how helping the subject has helped you, giving you an opportunity to give yourself great advice, reminding you of something that may have slipped your mind when you were caught in your own movie.

You may also notice how after the healing, you feel so much better than you did before the healing, and that even when you take back from the shelf all the stuff you put there just a short while before, it looks somehow different, and not so much of a problem any more. During the healing, you were healed as well, even though you did not enter the experience with that in mind.

Healing, then, has become a method of stimulating evolution, motivating us to experience love, and seeing the effects of love on the release of symptoms and the return of wholeness. Our desire to heal, and the act of healing, are after all both expressions of love. Besides, the value of healing another, as a form of self-therapy, has become evident. It has become a means of understanding the dynamics of creation and co-creation, exploring the nature of our being, and seeing how we can affect events in the external physical world. All this has happened with no external guru, no external master, no one but us deciding our own behavior and our own personal habits, and just doing what feels right for us, following our own conscience, and seeing with our own perceptions.

Through using healing as a teacher, we have also received a map of our own consciousness, and have seen the relationship between our consciousness and our body. We have learned how to use the tools with which we are able to explore our own consciousness to its deepest levels. We have gone beyond limiting ideas in a way that shows us how to apply the same principles in other parts of our lives. After all, if we are able to affect biological structure with our thoughts, what else can we do? Find out.

Anything can be healed.

CHAPTER 24

Responsibility and Helping Others

If you have accepted the idea that you are totally responsible for every-thing that happens in your life, and also for everything that happens in your body, and therefore for everything that happens in your conscious-ness, you must also have accepted the idea that no one else is responsible for you, or for the things that have happened in your life.

You have been faced with conditions, and it was you who decided how to respond to those conditions, and it was you who lived with the effects of having responded in that way.

In owning the responsibility for your own life, and in releasing others from that responsibility, it is important to recognize that others must be left with the responsibility for the things that have happened in their own lives, and in their own bodies. These have been the result of what they have chosen to put into their own consciousness, and the way they have chosen to respond to the conditions that have been presented to them in their own lives. In that way, you are not responsible for those others, or for what they have chosen to do with their own consciousness.

When parents are said to have responsibility for their children, they have agreed to accept that responsibility for the safety and wellbeing of those children, until the children are considered by society to be ready to assume the responsibility for themselves. The parents assume the respon-sibility for providing a home, and nourishment, and direction, and as much of a sense of well-being as they know how to provide.

Even here, however, the parents are not responsible for the way the child chooses to respond to its environment, nor for the ideas that the child chooses to accept into its consciousness. As a result of that, the child still creates its own reality, and is therefore still responsible for what happens in its life, and for what happens in its body, as the result of what it has chosen to put into its own consciousness.

Of course, there may be a possibility to offer some ideas that can help the child interact more successfully in the world, or release some symp-tom, but it remains the responsibility of the child to accept these ideas, or reject them, as the child chooses. If these ideas were offered with a sense of responsibility, then the presentation of the ideas has satisfied that responsibility, whether or not the child has chosen to accept those ideas.

Some people feel a sense of responsibility for sharing these ideas and services of healing with the society in which they find themselves. There, too, the sense of responsibility must end with the presentation of these possibilities, and not with whether or not the others have accepted these ideas or services.

We, as healers, know what can be done with these tools, and if others feel resistant, for any reason, to accept the help that is offered to them, we must know that any sense of responsibility has been satisfied, and that after that, the rest must remain the responsibility of the other. We can choose to offer our services where there is an openness and receptivity to them, and not waste our time and energy imposing these ideas where they are not welcome.

Some of us offer our services not from a sense of responsibility, but rather as an expression of love, because we know some way that others can feel much better, or even save their lives, with what is being offered. This expression of love doesn't come from a sense of obligation, but rather as a conscious choice motivated from within, and a true desire to see others happy and healthy. After all, the motivations for expressions of love must come from within, and not from an avoidance of guilt, if love is to make any sense as an evolutionary process.

In functioning as healers, we are implicitly offering our services to the society in which we find ourselves, whether that offering comes from a sense of responsibility to that society or as an expression of our love.

If it comes from a sense of responsibility, it can be very easy for us to feel thus responsible for every person in the world who is feeling ill or in pain, and in that way to feel bad for every person who is not feeling good. If we do that, however, we are then adding our own bad feelings to the total unhappiness of the world, making it an unhappier world. To create a world that is happier, we must begin with ourselves, by doing what is necessary to make ourselves happy.

We take the responsibility for developing ourselves as positive energy centers and can have a positive effect on the world around us, simply by being as happy and positive as we can be. One way to do this, of course, is by letting ourselves feel all of the love that it is possible for us to feel, and by letting that love radiate, affecting others in a positive way.

Then, when we see others who can benefit from what we do, we can see them with a sense of compassion and understanding, knowing that they have created their situation as the result of what they have been doing in their own consciousness. When we can do something for them, we are happy to do so, and happy to see them happy as a result. It is done as an expression of love, and although it is a responsible act, the motivation for doing it was not responsibility, but love. The motivating force was not the avoidance of a bad feeling, but rather a true desire to enhance the experience of another.

In that way, the true lesson of love was learned, and another level in the evolution of the individual, and of our planet, has been achieved. Love heals.

Anything can be healed.

CHAPTER 25

Love Heals

*When we wonder about the meaning of it all, the nature of the Universe,
the purpose of our being, the purpose of our evolution, and why we are
here, we may encounter in the esoteric philosophies the idea that we are
each and all gods and goddesses.*

Imagine being that. Being a god or goddess, when one is all that there is,
can be a very solitary experience. While we can experience being the creator
of the universe, containing all within, and constantly growing, expanding
infinitely, and loving our creation as an extension of our self, there are certain aspects of our own consciousness that are not accessible without considering co-creation and relating.

After all, can we be so chauvinistic as to believe that perhaps somewhere
out there, there may not be another god/goddess/all-that-there-is creating
their universe around them as we create ours around us? If so, how would
we communicate?

Jeffrey Love said it well in the preface to his book *The Quantum Gods:*

"The Quantum Gods are beings of infinite ability. Yet each of them exists
alone, unconscious of the existence of the others, and unable to manifest
as a creative being.

It is only through the creation of a common reality that the Quantum
Gods can attain consciousness of self and others. The Quantum Gods sign
a contract of intent in which they invest their very existence in the forma-
tion of a co-created reality. They are motivated to sign the contract out of
love—their desire to end their state of aloneness and to contact one another.
The contract is written with the pen of intentionality on the paper of space-
time in the ink of mass and energy. Their common reality is built of consciousness and a special condition of consciousness called matter. Matter
is the medium; being is the message.

...You and I are the Quantum Gods..." *

Then, the essential aspect of the contract underlying the creation of the
physical universe is one of love as its intention. It is love, therefore, that is
the cosmic "glue" holding it all together.

* Published by Samuel Weiser, New York, 1979.

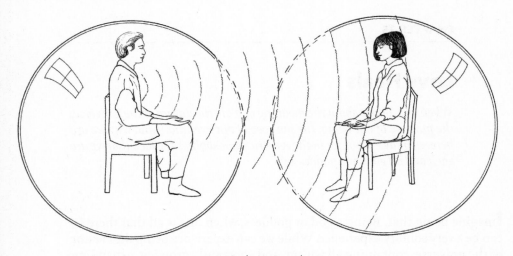

Love Radar Accepted

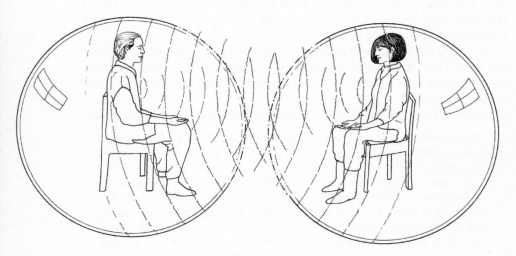

Love Radar Accepted and Returned

While we are each pure consciousness manifesting, the purpose of our manifestation is the evolution of our being, which must include love, the perception at the level of the Green Chakra, as an essential element.

From this level of perception, it is evident that everyone in the world is motivated by love, and sometimes reacting to the perception that it is not there. Nations guard their boundaries as an expression of love for their inhabitants. Other nations group together with others to create a sense of global community, again as an expression of love.

When we are born, love is necessary not only for our well-being, but also for our very survival. Without the sense of love and being wanted, children choose to not be born, or are born with parts of their energy systems impaired. We can say, in fact, that every symptom, every out-of-balance condition that can exist within the human energy system has, in fact, perceptions of lack of love as its underlying cause.

We know that every symptom represents tensions in the consciousness, and that these tensions represent different ways that we hold ourselves back from being who we really are. This is either a reaction to the perception that love is not there, or that it might be taken away if we allowed ourselves to be who we really are, because of someone else's ideas of what we "should" be doing. Either we feel not loved, or not worthy of love, or keep ourselves from being who we are because of the fear that love will be taken away.

Often, we play out scenarios in our lives that are repeats of what we have played before. The characters may be different, but the play is the same. When that happens, we seem bewildered, and ask ourselves, "Why am I seeing this movie again? Why am I living this scene again?"

To find the answer to that question, we can go back to the first time we saw that scene played out. That time, there was something incomplete about the scene. There was a missing ingredient. If that ingredient had been there, the scene would have been complete, and would not have left a question in our consciousness, and a sense of something not having been completed.

The missing ingredient is always the same. It is the perception that we are loved. The question in our consciousness that was unanswered was, "How can this be happening if I am loved?" The details may be different, but the basic question remains the same, whether the scenario is about desertion, or perceived wrongs, or misunderstandings. "If I were loved, this would not be happening. But it is happening. Therefore, I am not loved."

As long as this question is in our consciousness, we re-create the scenario in order to correct the erroneous perception, add the missing ingredient, and complete the scene in a way that leaves us with understanding, and the perception that the love was there, whether or not it had been perceived. There may have been perceived causes of the misperception, such as, "I'm not loved because I don't deserve love," or "It's because I did something wrong," or "I'm not good enough," etc. Our life will be lived from then on in a way that affirms the validity of those misperceptions, until we change our ideas.

To correct the problem, we can add the missing ingredient to the original scene, making it complete. We can add the perception that we were loved. It can be through replaying the scene from that point of view ("How must your father have felt having to leave you, if he really loved you?" "Oh, he must have felt really terrible."), or by sending out a "love radar," to see what comes back.

When the scene is replayed, adding the perception that we were indeed loved, something melts where there had been hardness, something feels softer, and we are able to let in the love we had for so long denied ourselves. Symptoms that had developed from the misperception can be released.

When we have difficulty creating in ourselves the perception that we are loved, "love radar" can help to show us that the love is there. To use it, we imagine ourselves in our own bubble, and send love to another whom we see in their bubble, and watch to see what happens as the love we are sending out reaches the other person. The other person may accept it quietly, or have difficulty letting it in, or be very happy about receiving it, and may, after having accepted it, choose to return it to us.

In sending the love, we can have a sense of when our love is being accepted, and when it is being returned. We can see it. Then, we know that the love is there, and we know it from what we have experienced. Even though it is a subjective experience, we will be able to validate this perception when we communicate with the other person on the physical level. If it is just too difficult for someone to create the perception on their own that the love is there, receiving a healing can help.

During the healing, it is important that we have absolutely no judgments or expectations concerning the subject. What we are left with when there are no judgments or expectations is acceptance and love, unconditional love. Within this environment of acceptance the subject is able to allow their own perceptions to be raised to the level of the heart, as well, releasing those erroneous perceptions that had been related to the creation of the symptom they have come to heal. They can feel the contact, and the love, and know that it is there.

And then the healing can happen.

Love heals.

Anything can be healed.

CHAPTER 26

Karma and Healing

Since we are all creators who have agreed to co-create a physical plane, we must have agreed to some system that holds everything together, some set of mechanics that reflects the unlimited and free nature of our being, as well as the nature of consciousness itself.

Karma is the name we have given to these mechanics. It is not a set of rules imposed from outside ourselves, but is merely the effect of what we do in our own consciousness. First of all, we must remember that the nature of our consciousness is to move us towards the completion of the pictures we choose to put into our own consciousness. When we have a goal and have put the picture of that goal into our consciousness, the fulfillment of the goal exists and we are moving towards it.

We can say that we have given our request to higher intelligence, whether we see this higher intelligence as something outside ourselves, or inside. Higher intelligence then gives us instructions, moment-to-moment, through the communication vehicle we call our intuition, or our instinct. Thus, our direction comes from *within* ourselves, in terms of doing what feels right to us, moment-to-moment.

At the same time, events in the outer world seem to be moving us in the same direction. These seem to be forces outside of ourselves, but they were set in motion by the picture or goal we have placed in our own consciousness. Thus, when certain things happen which seem to be directed by forces beyond our control yet at the same time are apparently in accord with what is supposed to happen, according to some kind of pattern and order, we say that it is karmic. Sometimes we also use the word *destiny* to describe the same force moving us in this way.

We can say, then, that one element of what we know as karma is that force that seems to be outside ourselves, propelling us towards the completion of our goals, yet set in motion by what we have done in our own consciousness. As we move towards this completion, two variables exist, namely, our actions and our perceptions. These, which we also decide, set in motion certain forces that seem to be outside of ourselves.

In terms of our actions, we say that what we do comes back to us. This is not meant in the sense of divine retribution, but rather simply as karmic mechanics, and as a means of communication. You see, there are many different ways of expressing love, and as we have mentioned earlier, the way that some people express their love is sometimes interpreted as the opposite of what was intended.

Fortunately, a protocol does exist that can help us to understand each other's sensitivities and preferences. If you want people to relate to you in a particular way, you can show them that way by example. Put out what you want back. Treat others as you would like them to treat you, and understand that others are treating you as they want to be treated.

It's as if they are saying, "This is how I like to have love expressed to me. If you want to express love to me, and this way of expressing it feels good for you to do, it is what feels good to me."

At the same time, they can be observing your actions, and understanding those as a demonstration of how you want love expressed to you, if it feels good for them to do it that way.

In terms of your relationship with the Universe, or whatever you choose to call the composite of energies that you perceive to be outside yourself, understand that the Universe is returning to you, through others, the energies and actions that have originated from you. While these energies are perceived to be outside yourself, they were set in motion by your actions, and they constitute a second element of what we call karma.

If it looks like divine retribution, consider the energies you have been putting out, because now you know what it feels like when they come back. Rather than continuing to create the same series of effects by continuing to put out the same energies, you can decide to create something different that will feel better when it returns to you. Thus, we can say that the "purpose" of this aspect of karma is understanding, and that once we achieve this understanding, we are released from the effects of that karma.

Of course, the positive aspects of your actions are also returned to you, in the sense of the Blue Chakra and the Green Chakra working together. As you flow along your path, expressing your love to others, and thereby satisfying their needs with no effort on their part at all, you find that your needs are met with no effort at all on your part, and also through an expression of the love of others. Thus, the love you put out comes back to you naturally.

In terms of your perceptions creating karma, we are talking of the way you choose to see others. We are all creators, each a soul, each a consciousness manifesting our Universe around us. In this way, we are all absolute equals. We all have the same equipment in our consciousness, and although some have manifested their abilities more than others have, we all have the same potential. We each have the same computer, although some have chosen to accept better programming.

From this point of view, we can say that when you look at the achievements of those you consider remarkable or extraordinary, they are only showing you an aspect of your own capabilities. What one can do, any can do. We are all equal, and in terms of our evolution, are all moving towards the Violet Chakra, representing unity. We are moving towards unity.

Unity does not exist in a hierarchical structure, but rather implies absolute equality. For one consciousness to be fully inside another in order to experience the other as itself with a sense of unity, the two must be absolutely equal. If you see someone as less than or greater than you, that is a misperception and must be corrected for the purposes of your evolution, and for the evolution of all.

If you see others as greater than you, you must understand it as a misperception. They have simply made you aware of your own capabilities, and have given you the tools for your growth, tools with which you can go beyond your own self-imposed limits. You have the ability to do what they have done, perhaps even better if you wish.

If you see others as less than you, your perceptions must also be adjusted. One way to do this is to "walk a mile in their shoes." The forces that move events in this direction seem to be coming from outside yourself, but they were set in motion by what you were doing in your own consciousness. This means of adjusting your perceptions is the third element of what we know as karma. We can see how its purpose is also understanding.

Thus, what we know as karma is made up of three elements:

1.   Moving us to the completion of our goals.
2.   Returning to us the effects of our actions.
3.   Adjusting our perceptions towards those of equality.

By looking at the events in our lives, those things that "happen to us," as being aspects of karma, we have a means of understanding certain things that did not make sense before. We can see a pattern and an order to things, and can release the tensions of misunderstanding that existed before.

We can see that what we know as karma is, at the same time, both totally personal and totally impersonal. It is personal in the sense that it reflects what we as individuals have chosen to do with our individual consciousness, and impersonal in the sense that it functions the same way for everyone. We can see that each of us is, at the same time, living the effects of past karma and building new karma, and sometimes it is difficult to tell which is which.

Since we each create and live our own karma, the idea that we can somehow "take on" the karma of another in any way demonstrates a misunderstanding of the nature of karmic mechanics. Some healers claim that certain symptoms cannot be healed because they are karmic. These healers are simply at the mercy of the effects of their own limiting ideas, and exporting their limitations in the form of some cosmic mystery. We believe that anything can be healed. The capacity to achieve this lies within each one of us.

From our point of view, all symptoms are karmic in that they are the effect of what people are doing in their own consciousness. This does not mean that they cannot be healed. If it was our karma to be ill, it can also be our karma to be healed, as was the case with me. If understanding is the purpose of karma, then that is in accord with our description of the relationship between the body and the consciousness.

When we develop a symptom, the symptom exists to give a message to us about some way of being that has been out of balance for us. We do to ourselves literally what we have been doing figuratively.

When we understand the message that our body has been giving and make the necessary adjustments in our way of being, the symptom has no further reason for existing and can be released. It is for this reason, remember, that it is important for us as healers to communicate the inner cause of the outer symptom, as an integral part of the healing.

It is also important for us to remember that we are unlimited in our consciousness, and that any idea that limits us is, by its nature, invalid. We have an unlimited ability to heal anything. If there is some idea that gives us a reason to believe that we do not have the ability to perform this important spiritual service, we can replace this idea with another that gives us the means to go beyond this perceived limit.

We know that anything can be healed.

CHAPTER 27

Questions and Answers

Q. Must the healer know what the problem is before the healing can happen?

With the Body Mirror System, the healer is able to see whether or not a subject's energy system is in balance. In that way, it is not necessary for the healer to be aware of what the problem is before looking into the energy system. If you are aware that there is a problem before looking, you can focus attention in a particular area. If not, you will probably see it anyway. Of course, it depends on the depth to which you are looking.

When you take your car to the mechanic, he does not need to know what the problem is beforehand in order to fix it. His own examination of the car will reveal what needs to be done. Often, in fact, problems are healed that the subject did not communicate to the healer, nor even think of, but which the subject recognized when the healer described them.

It should be emphasized here that healers do not diagnose illnesses. They merely see the state of balance of an energy system. They can see that there is tension in a particular part of the consciousness, but that tension may manifest in a number of different ways. If a healer sees shadows, for example, it would not be appropriate to say that the subject has cancer.

In the same way, healers may not tell subjects that they no longer have cancer. They may only comment that they no longer see evidence of it in the subject's energy system. Thus, healers do not impose themselves in areas of legality reserved for members of the medical profession.

Q. What causes birth defects, and what do we need to know in order to heal them?

According to our model, everything begins in the consciousness. This is as true for a baby, even a fetus, as it is for an adult. As adults, we decide how to respond to conditions in our environment, and sometimes these conditions are difficult. Babies do the same.

When someone speaks of birth defects, the first question to ask is when the symptom was detected. Often, something is discovered some time after the actual process of birth, but described as a birth defect. If a symptom was detected at two years old, for example, the relevant question is, "What was happening in this being's life at that time? What difficult circumstances presented themselves at that time?" We might then discover that at that age, another child was born in the family, or that the parents decided to divorce.

We might learn that a child had been born prematurely and kept in an incubator for two months, after which it was discovered to be blind. Was it really a birth defect, or is there a possibility that the baby was born with sight, but then reacted to being put in an environment of isolation, with little or none of the contact that was so important for it at that time?

What is of primary importance is that the baby feels in contact with its parents, and welcomed into their world.

For example, a baby in Florida was born with a tumor at the base of its spine, in that part of the energy system that we associate with its relationship with its mother. When I spoke with the mother, she explained that the tumor, according to the doctors, had begun to grow in her sixth month of pregnancy. Naturally, I asked her what was happening in her life as a prospective mother during her sixth month of pregnancy. She explained that she and her husband had had a terrible fight. He had left, and it did not seem that he was going to return. I asked her how she felt about having a baby if he did not return, and she told me that she did not want to be a single mother. If he did not come back, she would not want to have the baby.

When she made that decision, the tumor began to grow inside the child. It was as if the child had been aware of everything that had been happening. From its point of view, it first felt itself loved and wanted, and then not wanted, without knowing why. It was as if the baby was saying, "If you don't really want me, I don't really want to be there." The parents reconciled and decided that they wanted this child. When it was born with the tumor, it was given a 50% chance of survival. It was as if the baby had decided to take a chance on coming into the world, but was not yet certain. The baby received enormous amounts of love and attention, and the tumor was healed.

We can look at each of the participants in this event to see how each created this situation. Thus, we can see how the mother did not want to bring a child into her life if there was no partner, and when she decided that, circumstances began to manifest in that direction. We can, of course, say the same about the father.

Our main focus as healers is on the consciousness of the person experiencing the physical symptom in order to understand how the symptom was created, and thus how to heal it. We can see, however, that counseling other members of the immediate family can sometimes be very helpful in providing additional levels of understanding.

Q. Isn't it true that sometimes accidents just happen?

Our model is always based on the idea that everything begins in the consciousness. When we create tension in our consciousness with a decision we make regarding a response to conditions facing us, we know that the tension can manifest on the physical level if there is sufficient intensity, or if the tension is there over a long enough period of time. The symptom, however, must manifest according to physical cause-and-effect reality. There must be a physical cause.

We know that we have an inner guidance system that we call intuition, or instinct. If we do not listen at this level, we feel more and more emotions that do not feel good as we continue to move in a certain direction. If we still don't listen, we receive the message at the next level of communication, which is the physical body. We can then create a symptom that gives us a message. It reflects the idea that we each create our reality.

If our intuition is always accurate, we can ask ourselves what guided us to be in a particular place at a particular time where an accident was about to happen. If the result was some kind of symptom, we can say that the end result was the real intention. The event happened in order to create the symptom, in order for us to receive a message from our body that we had not been paying attention to at the level of intuition or emotions.

Thus, when there was a need for the message at the physical level, Spirit guided us, through our intuition (newly adjusted), to circumstances that could provide the symptom. If the accident had not happened, the symptom would have had to be created another way, through a disease or a pinched nerve, for example.

Group accidents are co-created, also. According to circumstances, all of the people involved had made a decision to be there, or had been guided in that direction. Individuals who had changed something in their consciousness just before the event tell stories of following a "hunch" and not getting on a certain plane that later crashed, or being prevented by circumstances (such as waking up late or car trouble) from being involved in that group event destined to be a disaster. Was that just luck, or coincidence? Or was there a reason?

There are no accidents, and no coincidences. There is a pattern and order to the universe and the way it manifests. While some people prefer to stand in awe of the mysteries of the universe, and to be impressed with the idea that it is not possible for humans to understand its workings, we can see from the level of the Indigo Chakra how the physical world manifests each event according to each of the consciousnesses involved in that event.

This is why we say that by looking at the manifestation of events in the physical world, we can then see what has been happening in the consciousness of each of the individuals involved in those events. One reflects the other. The physical world reflects the consciousness.

Q. What is death? What is it like to die?

Death is the ultimate transformation, and it happens to at least most people (there are some stories about exceptions, such as the Count Saint Germain and Babaji). Considering its universality, it is amazing that so little is known about it.

We are each a spirit occupying a body. Despite the degree to which we have identified with the body that serves as our vehicle, nothing changes the truth that who we are is the being within. At some point, we leave the body, and also the personality we had developed while in it, and we return to the level of being we identify as spirit, which is just the deeper aspect of our consciousness. We let go of certain attitudes, ideas, and values with which we have identified, and we experience another point of view. It is what we consider more evolved, more spiritual. It also feels much better.

Because many people do not understand the process called death, and have no idea of what lies beyond, they are afraid. They are not aware that they will continue to experience something.

Normally, when we leave our body, we experience something like falling through a tunnel, at the end of which there is a light. This is the passage out of the body, and the process of returning to whatever can be considered the Source.

Commonly, we are met on the other side by some sort of being or a welcoming committee. This might be a relative, or spiritual leader, or friends. They are there to help re-orient the recently arrived spirit. While the letting go and emotional acceptance of death might be difficult for some people, the passage through the tunnel and welcome into the light are universally described as a beautifully joyous transcendent experience.

As healers, our function is to help the people with whom we are working with whatever they have decided to do. If on a deep level, someone does not really want to continue with their life, the form of the healing may be for them to feel okay about their decision to leave their body, and to help them with understanding the passage. In this way, the love and the help we offer are unconditional.

When healers help with the passage, they can do this from the outside, or from the inside. That is, they can choose to direct the attention of the subject while not being directly involved in the experience, or they can be in contact with the subject's spirit and go along for the ride.

When directing the experience from the outside, the healer can reassure the subject about the quality of the experience, and direct the subject's attention towards the light, and to the waiting welcoming being or beings. Offering this love and support helps to make the experience much easier, and a joyous one.

When going along for the ride, the healer feels their consciousness linked with that of the subject. The experience can be initiated by either the subject or by the healer. In this kind of experience, the benefit to the person making the passage is that they need not be alone in the experience. Most people make the passage alone, and for someone afraid of the aloneness of the experience, being accompanied is a spiritual service of inestimable value.

As the subject experiences the initial vertigo of the experience, the healer feels the same thing, like falling into a black hole, or fainting, except that the subject continues to consciously experience what is happening. When the two consciousnesses are linked, it may also be the healer who initiates the experience, dropping down into their own consciousness, while noticing that the subject is responding in a way that shows they are experiencing the same thing. If machines were monitoring the subject, the slowing of the machines would also show that the subject is responding as we have described.

There is no need for the healer to fear the experience. Those who accompany always return afterwards, and their own spiritual evolution is enhanced, as well. They are also able to use their own experience as a basis for communicating to other people what happens during the process. That, too, is a service.

Healing has many forms.

Anything can be healed.

Energy Exercises and Meditation

CHAPTER 28

Energy Exercises

Preliminaries

These exercises are intended to demonstrate, through your experience, principles discussed in this book that are applicable to the technology of healing, as well as to your ability to feel and direct energy, and thus function as a healer.

Even though these exercises can be done alone, they can be even more interesting if you do them with another person, reading the instructions aloud as you both follow them, and discussing between you what you experience. If you are alone at this time, consider repeating the exercises another time with a friend present, for an even deeper experience.

First, place this book on a table or a stand where you can continue to read it without holding it. In this way, you can free your hands, so that you can follow the instructions. While this will be easiest if you are seated, it is not absolutely necessary if you can keep your attention on the instructions as you continue to follow them.

Exercise A—Basic Energy Exercise: Feeling the Energy

Now, place your hands on the table or (even better) your lap, with your palms facing upward. Put your attention on the palms of your hands, and on the surface of the skin on the palms of your hands. Feel the air against the skin there. You may be aware of the temperature of the air, or the movement of the air, or the pressure of the air. Spend some moments with this, feeling it more and more.

As you keep your attention there, become more and more aware of the skin that the air is touching. Soon, you will be aware of another sensation, perhaps like a tingling or vibration, something different from your ordinary experience. It may be subtle at first, but as you direct your attention to it

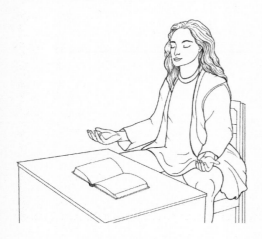

Preparing to Feel Energy

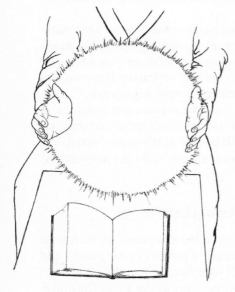

Holding Ball of Energy

more and more, you can feel it becoming more and more definite.

We can give a name to this sensation. We can call it energy. Imagine that something called energy is flowing through your hands, vibrating the membrane of the skin as it passes through on its way out. Can you imagine it to be that, which you are experiencing now? Imagine that what you are feeling is energy flowing through your hands. Imagine that what you feel is your hands glowing with energy. Feel the energy radiating from your hands.

Keeping the sensitivity on your hands, place them facing each other about 45 centimeters (18 inches) apart, and move them slowly towards each other and then away from each other, back and forth. Notice that your hands feel different when they are moving towards each other than when they are moving apart.

You can imagine that there is a ball of energy between your hands, and that as you bring your hands towards each other, you are compressing the ball, and "packing" more energy into it, making it more dense. It's like packing a snowball, but this is an energy ball. Soon, you are able to feel the outline, the surface, of this ball of energy, and you can hold this ball, maintaining the sensitivity of your hands.

If you are working with another person, face each other, each of you holding your own ball of energy, and move your hands in a way that allows you to feel your partner's energy. For example, you may move your hands so that one of yours is between your partner's, moving up and down through their energy field. Notice the sensations you experience on your hands as you do this. Your partner, of course, can be doing the same thing at the same time. Spend some moments doing this.

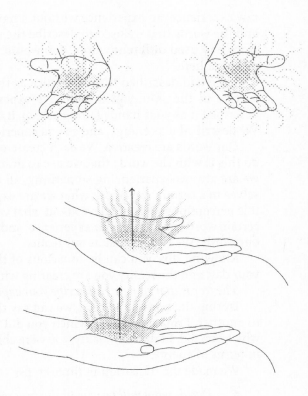

Afterwards, relax your hands, and examine what you have experienced. Some people describe the experience by using words such as "heat" or "cold," "electricity" or "magnetism," a "flow" or a "density." All of these words can be recognized as different forms of energy, or different aspects of energy, in the same way that there are different aspects of energy coming from a light bulb. Some would describe these as "light," others as "heat," and still others as "a magnetic field." We can see that all would be correct. They are all different aspects of the energy that is there.

Energy Vibrations

Whatever you felt, we can say that it is the sensation that tells you that you are feeling energy. Some people notice that when they feel another's energy, the sensations are different from when they feel their own, yet still something that they can relate to as energy.

Several things happened during this exercise. You started with just a

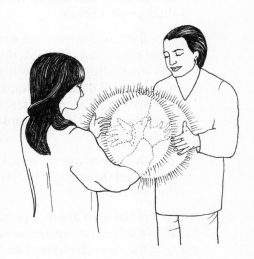

Partners Feeling Energy

raw experience, an experience without a name. Then, we called it energy, and the words that we used to describe the experience created the reality. If we had used different words, you would have experienced something different here.

If we had described the experience as the blood flowing beneath the surface of the skin, you would have experienced it as that. If we had described it as your hands falling asleep, it would have been that for you. We described it as energy, and so you experienced it as that.

Our words are creative. We each create our reality; one of the ways we do this is with the words that we use to describe our experience. After all, we are always experiencing something, all day long, and we talk to ourselves in a certain way about what we are experiencing. With all the possible perceptions we could have about what we are experiencing, we choose certain words to describe our experience, and energize that perception with our words. We choose that as our reality.

Knowing this, you can be conscious of the words that you use during your day, and the reality you are creating with these words.

The words that you use to describe your experience create your reality.

During the exercise you did, we can say that you went from one reality to another. From a reality in which you did not feel energy to a reality in which you did. In the new reality, you were able to describe your experiences in terms of energy.

We made the transition in three steps:

1.   *Decide what will be true in the new reality.* We decided what would be true in the new reality. We decided that you were going to feel something in your hands.

2.   *Encourage the perception that it's happening now.* While the first step could come from this book, the second step had to come from you. That was you reaching for the way the words made sense. Perhaps you said to yourself, "I think I feel something now. Perhaps that's what this book is describing. Yes, now I feel it more and more." You encouraged the perception that it was happening now, giving yourself reasons to believe in the process.

3.   *Decide that now it's true.* Finally, you could decide, "Now, it's true. Now, I feel the energy. Now, I can feel my partner's energy. Now, I'm in the new reality."

If you worked with another person, you might also recognize that what began as a subjective experience was then able to be experienced by another being in the external physical world, making it a shared experience, objective, and real.

Healing works like that, too. The perception of the healing, which begins in the consciousness of the healer as a subjective experience, can then be experienced in the external physical world by others. Thus it works and accomplishes something for them.

When we prepare for a healing, we always begin by placing our hands in the same position, on a table or on our legs with the palms facing upwards. We then recall and re-create the sensation of energy in our hands. In this way, we are able to use our hands as a biofeedback device, to give us the feedback that we are in a particular state of consciousness.

A biofeedback device works with the idea that in different states of consciousness, biological functions change. There are changes in the breathing rate, perspiration rate, blood pressure, heartbeat, etc. When the biological functions measured by the device show that we are at the state of consciousness in which we are interested, the machine gives us feedback. A bell rings, or a needle moves, or a light flashes.

The machine is saying to us, "You are now in the state of consciousness in which you are interested." When we become familiar with the state of consciousness, we do not need the machine to tell us that we are there.

With biofeedback, we may be seeking an alpha or theta state of consciousness. With the process we use, we are seeking the state of consciousness in which we feel energy. Since we heal with energy, it is the state of consciousness in which a healing can happen.

As long as the sensation is in your hands, you are in a perfect state of consciousness to successfully perform a healing. During the healing, if the sensation stops, you must stop, and re-establish the sensation before you continue the healing. You can create the sensation whenever you wish.

Sometimes, the sensation may come without your having called for it, but it still means the same thing. It means that you are in a state of consciousness in which you are able to function as a healer. It may be that in a short while, someone will tell you that they do not feel well in some way, and then you will know why the sensations appeared. It was for this person's healing, if they are open to that. You can offer your services as a healer, leaving the other person to decide whether or not to participate in the healing process with you. If so, go for it. If not, leave it alone.

Because we always start the healings with this position, we have a special name for it. We call it the Healing Starting Position.

Always remember that *anything can be healed.*

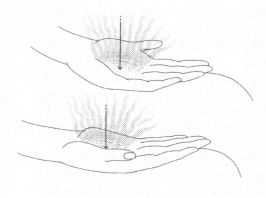

Energy Flowing In

Exercise B—Directing Energy

Now, create the sensation once more in your hands, by just focusing on the sensations on the surface of the skin on the palms of your hands, remembering the sensations in order to recreate them.

This time, we will describe the experience with different words. Imagine that what you feel is energy flowing in through your hands, vibrating the skin on the way in. You can imagine that your hands are like radar receivers, sensitive to energy, and that the space around you is filled with energy. There are radio waves and television waves, x-rays and gamma waves, mental energy, sexual energy, light and sound energy, heat energy, love energy, healing energy—an ocean of energy—and you can feel this energy coming into your hands.

Feel the energy traveling in through your hands, traveling up your arms, and into your body. Feel this energy charging your batteries. Feel yourself being energized throughout. Feel yourself becoming clearer, more centered, more of whatever you would imagine to be the benefits of this energy entering you. Spend some time with this, filling yourself with this energy, and finally feeling yourself glowing with this energy over the entire surface of your body, shining like a light bulb.

Now, redirect your attention to the palms of your hands again, and the surface of the skin. This time, we are going to describe the sensations in a different way again. Decide that what you feel now is the sensation of your hands glowing with energy. Feel the energy radiating from your hands again, as you did during the first exercise.

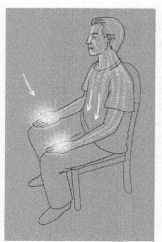

Drawing Energy In

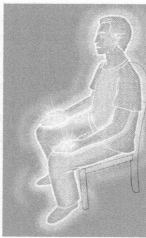

Filling with Energy

As you feel the energy glowing from your hands, we can give it yet another name. We can call it White Light. You can imagine that the sensation you experience is that of White Light radiating from your hands, and then it's easy to imagine the glow as a White Light. We heal with White Light. Spend some moments experiencing this, and then relax your hands and continue reading.

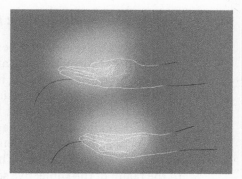

Hands Glowing with White Light

When you decided that the energy was flowing into your hands, you could feel it moving in that direction, and experience its effects. When you decided that the energy was flowing out from your hands, not only were you able to feel it like that, another person was able to experience it, as well. You did not have to force the energy out, or suck it in. There was no effort involved. You only had to decide which way the energy would move, and then feel it moving in that direction, using the three steps mentioned in Exercise A:

1. *Decide what will be true in the new reality.*
2. *Encourage the perception that it's happening now.*
3. *Decide that now it's true.*

From what you have experienced so far, you know that you are able to feel energy. You know it because you have experienced doing that. You also know that you are not only able to detect energy, but also direct energy, because you have done that as well. This energy is always flowing through you, and you are aware now that your consciousness can direct this energy. In fact, we believe that you have always been directing this energy with your consciousness. We are beings of energy, and when we block the flow of this energy with sufficient intensity, the result is some kind of symptom.

All symptoms, then, can be described as merely blocked energy. Since you have the ability to direct energy, you are able to unblock the energy wherever it has been blocked, in yourself or others. When you do that, the healing happens. When we look at things in this way, it is apparent that anything can be healed. You can heal anything. After all, didn't a certain well-known healer from the past say that what he could do, you could do, and maybe even better? Don't you believe he was right?

Anything can be healed.

Exercise C—Seeing Energy: Auras

With this exercise, you will be increasing the subtlety of your subjective experiences and experiencing alternative visual realities. Please remember that the subjective senses are, by their nature, subjective. That is, they are happening in your own consciousness, and it may feel as though you are imagining them. If this is true for you, you do not need to use the subjectivity of the experience as a reason to invalidate the experience.

In the scientific world, we are taught that there are things that are real, and those that are imagined. This implies that what is imagined is not real. In the realm of the subjective senses, however, we can recognize that even though something feels imagined, that makes it no less real. In entering alternative visual realities, you will be using the familiar three steps:

1.   *Decide what will be true in the new reality.* Decide that you will see something different.
2.   *Encourage the perception that it's happening now.* Give yourself reasons to believe that your experience is showing that it is happening now. You are beginning to see something happen now.
3.   *Decide that now it's true.* Decide that now you are seeing something, even if it feels like you are imagining it, and describe to yourself the visual experience that is happening, and what it looks like to you.

First, with your hands resting in your lap close to but not touching each other, re-create the experience in your hands during Exercise B, Directing Energy. Feel your hands glowing with energy. Decide that they are glowing with White Light. Do it now, before reading further.

Next, watch your hands in your lap while you are deciding that they are glowing with White Light, and imagine that you see the glow. Some people see it as something like heat waves that rise from the sidewalk on a hot summer day, while others see it more as a glow of white energy, but decide that you will see something that you will be able to relate to the experience of White Light, which is glowing from your hands.

You can do it now.

If it felt like your eyes were playing tricks with you, that's all right. All we are interested in here is a visual experience. Whatever it was, and even if you thought it was an optical illusion, it was what you experienced, and if you were asked to, you could describe or draw a picture of what it looked like. For our purposes, that's perfect.

The next step can be done alone while looking into a mirror, or while facing a partner, and looking into the eyes of the face before you. If you have not been accustomed to seeing energy, you should know that it is easier if the room is dimly lit, and if there is a uniform background behind the subject.

Whether you are looking at a partner or your own reflection, it is best if you look not at the surface of the eyes, but rather behind them, or deeply into them, to the being who is there. While your primary attention is there, allow your secondary attention, your peripheral vision, to notice what it looks like around the face that you see before you.

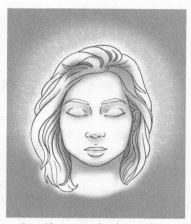

Face Glowing with White Light

Remember the visual experience you had with your hands, and watch for something similar. You may see changes in the face before you. It might take on other forms, or become other faces, and this is a natural and normal phenomenon for anyone doing the same thing, exposing the same spiritual dimensions. Just now, keep your attention on the glow you see that you can relate to as the aura.

Some people see it as a glow or a light, while some also experience pale pastel colors. The colors seen can be related to the chakra colors, and can show where the person is in their consciousness in that moment. For example, if they are glowing emerald green, they can be said to be in the state of consciousness we relate to the Green Chakra, and so on.

Do the exercise now for at least one or two minutes, as described, and if you are working with a partner, have a communication afterward about what was seen. Perhaps you will find that if you each saw colors, you will be able to relate the colors that were seen to what was being experienced in the consciousness of the other.

If you did not see colors, describe to each other what you did see. You can repeat the exercise several times, while holding different states of consciousness, to see how the visual experience changes. For example, you can do the exercise while imagining you are glowing with White Light, or with particular colors, or while feeling energy in your heart, or while feeling angry about something, or while thinking analytically, and see what different visual experiences present themselves.

With practice, you will be easily able to create this experience at will, and use it as another level of communication available to you, which shows you what is happening in the consciousness of the beings around you. With the realization of their visibility, you will realize your own state of being is always visible, and if you have been putting a lot of energy into pretending to be invisible, you will be able to drop it, as a waste of time, and put your energy to better use in another way.

Anything can be healed.

CHAPTER 29

Chakra Meditation

With this experience, you will be directing your attention to each of the chakras in turn, first by focusing on physical sensations, and then by using your imagination, your ability to create images, to create the experience of colors there. There is no difference between imagination and visualization, except for the fact that most people believe more in their ability to imagine than in their ability to visualize. They know that even children can imagine things, but visualization... well, that's another thing.

While you will be asked to imagine certain colors in certain places, you may have impressions of other colors. If this happens, just notice what the other colors are that you are having an impression of, and then release them, and replace them with the proper color. You will be able to do this by imagining that you are shining lights of the proper color on the chakra, or painting it the proper color, or imagining something of the proper color there. Finally, you will be able to create an impression of the proper colors in the proper places, and experience the effects of that.

If there were impressions of colors different from those asked for, this will show you something about what was happening in that portion of your consciousness. You will be able to consult the Color Language Reference Guide (Appendix 3) and see what the colors that you saw mean in terms of our model of wholeness, and how the description found in the chart matches what you know to have been happening in your own consciousness.

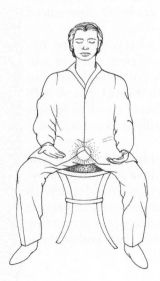

Now, find a comfortable position, and do the meditation as follows:

First, direct your attention to your perineum, and to the physical sensations you experience there. Feel something. Decide that what you are feeling is energy, and then decide that this energy is glowing red. If you have an impression of another color, notice what it is, and then release it, and make it red. Have a final impression of a clear red ball of energy where you know your Red Chakra to be. Hold your attention there, doing that, for some moments.

Next, move your attention up about ten centimeters (four inches), to the middle of your abdomen, and to the physical sensations you experience there. Feel something, and decide that what you are feeling is energy.

Then, decide that this energy is glowing orange. If you have an impression of another color, just notice what it is, and then release it, and change the colour to orange. Finally, have an impression of a clear orange ball of energy where you know your Orange Chakra to be, and hold your attention there, doing that for some moments.

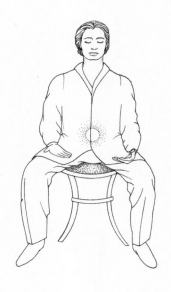

Now, move your attention to your solar plexus. Be aware of sensations there. Feel something, and decide that what you are feeling is energy. Then, decide that this energy is glowing yellow. If you have an impression of another color, just notice what it is, and then change it, and make it yellow. Have a final impression of a clear yellow ball of energy glowing in your Yellow Chakra, and hold that experience for some moments.

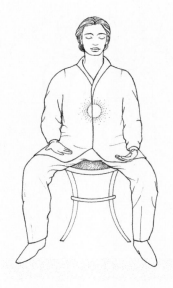

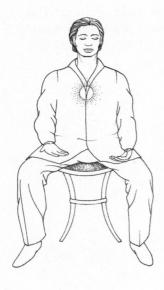

Now, move your attention to the center of your chest, where you know your Green Chakra to be. Be aware of sensations there. Feel something, and decide that what you feel is energy, and that it is glowing emerald green. If you have an impression of another color, just notice what it is, and then release it, and make it emerald green. Hold the impression of a clear emerald green ball of energy in your Green Chakra for some moments, experiencing it.

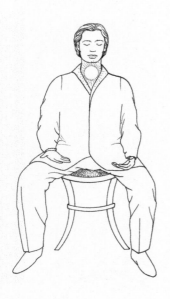

Now, move your attention to the base of your throat. Be aware of sensations there. Feel something there where you know your Blue Chakra to be, and decide that what you are feeling is energy, and that it is glowing blue, sky blue. If you have an impression of another color there, just notice what it is, and change it. Decide that now, it is sky blue. Hold the final impression of a clear sky blue ball of energy in your Blue Chakra for some moments.

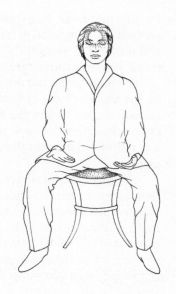

Next, place your attention on the center of your forehead. Be aware of sensations there, feel something where you know your Indigo Chakra to be, and decide that what you are feeling is energy. Decide that it is glowing indigo, midnight blue. If you have an impression of another color there, just notice what it is, and release it. Change it. Decide that now it is indigo, and hold for some moments an impression of an indigo ball of energy in your Indigo Chakra.

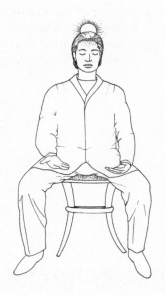

Now, move your attention to the top of your head. Be aware of sensations there, where you know your Violet Chakra to be. Feel something, and decide that what you are feeling is energy. Then, decide that this energy is glowing violet, the color of amethyst. If you have an impression of another color, just notice what it is, and change it. Make it violet, and hold a final impression for some moments of a violet ball of energy glowing in the Violet Chakra.

Finally, just relax, and notice the state of being you experience after the meditation, compared to how you felt before the experience. No doubt, you will notice how you feel better in some way, and you will therefore understand, through your experience, the benefits of this meditation.

The meditation not only helps you to re-center yourself when you need to, but also gives you an inventory of what has been happening in your consciousness just before the experience, a picture of where you are. You can expect that after the work you have done on yourself with this meditation, any out-of-balance conditions have been corrected, or improved to some degree.

The inventory of where you are is the result of the analysis of the colors that were seen in the various chakras, as shown in the Color Language Reference Guide chart previously mentioned. If you saw only the proper colors in areas that you know to have been out of balance, such as those areas associated with particular physical symptoms you have been experiencing, you will know that your view of yourself was not reflecting what was real, but rather what you wanted it to be. It is necessary that your view of where you are in any moment is without any element of self-deception, or you will not have the mechanism available to improve something that the deeper part of you knows to be out of balance.

Know yourself and what is true for you. Accept this. That's the starting point for everything else.

Remember that anything can be healed.

Appendices

The Chakra Healing Guide

The Red Chakra

Also known as: Root Chakra, Security Center, *Muladhara.*

Location: The perineum, the point between the anus and the sex organs.

Parts of the body: The parts of the body associated with this chakra include the lymph system and the skeleton system (teeth and bones), the prostate gland in men, the sacral plexus, and the parts of the body and functions within the body controlled by the sacral plexus. These include the bladder and the elimination system, and the lower extremities (the legs, and the different parts of the legs – the feet, ankles, etc.).

Note: When we say that this chakra is associated with a particular system, we mean that something that affects that entire system can be traced to tension in this chakra. For example, something that affects the entire skeleton system, like systemic arthritis, can be traced to tension in the Red Chakra, but a broken arm, which is a skeletal problem in a particular part of the body, rather than throughout the entire body, would be traced instead to tension in the chakra controlling that particular part of the body, in this case, the arm, and that would be related to the Blue Chakra.

Within the endocrine system, the Red Chakra is associated with the adrenal glands. Technically, the secretions of the adrenal glands can be associated with

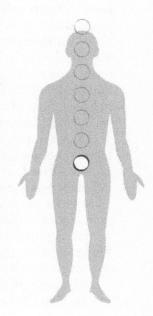

both the Red Chakra and the Yellow Chakra, but the fact that they are triggered by a threat to survival shows their primary association to be with the Red Chakra.

Sense: The physical sense associated with this chakra is the sense of smell, the basic sense associated with survival. Therefore, the organ associated with the sense of smell, the nose, is also associated with the Red Chakra.

Consciousness: The Red Chakra is associated with the parts of consciousness concerned with security, survival, and trust—feeling safe and secure. For most people, the parts of their lives concerned with security have to do with their relationship with money, their home, and their job. Being able to feel "at home" as well as being present in the here and now, are also associated with this chakra.

Element: The element associated with the Red Chakra is earth. The Red Chakra can therefore be said to reflect, among other things, our relationship with the earth, or how we feel about being on the earth.

The Red Chakra also reflects our relationship with our mother. In the traditional family structure, the mother provides the nourishment and a safe space for her child. The baby nursing at its mother's breast makes certain decisions about the way things are ("There's always abundance," or "There's never enough," or "You have to fight to get what you want," etc.). The relationship the baby has with its mother then sets the pattern for that person's relationship with everything that represents security (home, and job, and money as security).

When we experience a sense of separation from our mother, not perceiving ourselves to be loved or nourished by her, we cut off our own roots with those perceptions, and create a blockage at the level of the Root Chakra, or Red Chakra. The effect, the way we experience this in our consciousness, is to have a filter of insecurity or fear through which we see the world, until we can again open to allow ourselves to be nourished by her love.

Other symptoms experienced by someone without roots can be not having a home, not feeling at home, not being grounded, not having their perceptions based on their personal experience in the physical world, and difficulty being present in the here and now.

When a person is looking at the world through the Red Chakra, the motivations in that moment have to do with security, survival, feeling safe, or meeting material needs. It can also be about seeking nourishment for the inner being, that is, not food, but rather that which gives you, the person inside your body, a sense of solidity and satisfaction.

When our primary motivating force in life is security, or survival, we can say that the Red Chakra is our home during that part of our life, and that from that chakra, we move our consciousness to the other chakras, depending on what is being thought about or felt in a particular moment. (The primary motivating force is defined as the basis from which all decisions are made, and as that which motivates the individual.)

When the Red Chakra is in its clear state, individuals are able to feel safe and at home, solid and grounded. They are able to feel present in their physical body, present in the here and now where they are, and able to function in the physical material world. They are able to trust their perceptions, and in general, do not have a problem with trust as a process.

Tension in the Red Chakra is experienced emotionally as insecurity. Additional tension there is experienced as fear. More tension there is experienced as a threat to survival. When the tension continues for a period of time, or to an extreme of intensity, the person creates a symptom in a part of the body or a function within the body associated with or controlled by the Red Chakra.

Therefore, any out-of-balance condition or symptom affecting parts of the body or functions within the body associated with the Red Chakra is reflecting tension in the person's consciousness in the Red Chakra concerning security, survival, trust, willingness or ability to be nourished, and/or the relationship with the mother.

It must be emphasized here that the mother's actions or way of being have nothing to do with the person's symptoms. It is, rather, the way the individual has chosen to respond to the conditions in life that have resulted in the stress and tension. Two children in the same family, for example, may be experiencing the same external conditions, but responding differently, to their situation, so that one experiences symptoms, and the other does not.

We do not say that certain conditions cause certain symptoms. Rather, we say that given certain symptoms, we can understand the conditions that the person was experiencing with stress. If there is a problem with the Red Chakra on one side of the body or another, we examine that in terms of the polarity of the will side and the emotional side, or the male side and the female side. (As was previously mentioned, for those who were born right-handed, their right side is their will side. For those born left-handed, their left side is their will side.)

Thus, a problem with the will leg can be interpreted in terms of the effects of the symptoms. If someone needs to be supported (with crutches or a cane, for example), we can say that that describes what the person has been doing in their consciousness—needing and soliciting support for decisions, and not trusting their will. Such people decide to do something, but do not act on it until they have received enough support from others affirming that they have made the right decision.

If we describe the affected or blocked leg as the male leg, this can represent blocked trust (the aspect of the Red Chakra) in a male. If it is a male whose leg is affected, we can also describe the symptoms as reflecting nontrust in himself as a man.

If it is the emotional leg that is affected, we can say that this represents tension in the foundation of the emotions, or emotional dependency on someone else. Those affected make decisions designed to hold onto someone, rather than deciding what is best for themselves. Or, they can have experienced an emotional shock regarding Red Chakra issues of money, home, or job.

If we describe the leg as the female leg, it can represent blocked trust in a female. If it is a female whose female leg is affected, we can say that it can represent not trusting herself as a woman.

We can also read the symptoms in terms of what the person needs in order to return to balance. For example, if the person's leg does not bend, and that affects mobility, we can say that they need, for their healing, more flexibility and freedom of movement.

If there is a problem with the kidneys, even though they are located at the level of the solar plexus, we consider them in their roles concerning the elimination system. Their location at the level we associate with perceptions of power or freedom (the Yellow Chakra) can be combined with the level we associate with trust (the Red Chakra), and we can read the symptom as insecurity concerning power (perceived lack of power, making oneself appear helpless) or as insecurity about freedom (perceived lack of freedom, feeling restricted).

We can also consider the function of the kidneys in reading the symptoms. The kidneys cleanse the blood of toxins. The blood represents the heart, or perceptions of love, and the toxins represent attitudes that interfere with the person's perceptions of love. These have reached an intensity that threatens personal survival, and there is need for change. Such people need to allow the love around them to nourish them, releasing the attitudes that threaten their survival.

Allergies to substances we associate with mothering, such as milk and dairy products, or those that we associate with the earth, such as wheat products, and those allergies that affect the nose, such as hay fever, all reflect tensions in the Red Chakra, and in people's relationship with their mother, in which they have been giving themselves reasons to keep themselves from being nourished. When these attitudes change, the symptoms can be released.

Anything can be healed.

The Orange Chakra

Also known as: Sensation Center, Spleen Chakra, Hara, *Svadhistana*.

Location: The center of the abdomen.

Parts of the body: The parts of the body associated with this chakra include the reproductive system, the sexual organs, the lumbar plexus, and the parts of the body and functions within the body controlled by the lumbar plexus, as well as those in the region of the abdomen.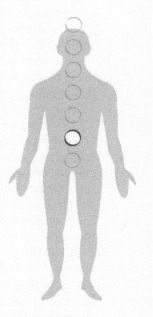

The endocrine glands associated with this chakra are the gonads (the testes and the ovaries).

Sense: The physical sense associated with this chakra is the sense of taste, and the appetite. Therefore, the tongue as the organ of taste can be said to be associated with the Orange Chakra. This chakra is also associated with that aspect of the sense of touch having to do with sensations.

Consciousness: The Orange Chakra is associated with the parts of the consciousness concerned with food and sex, as well as with having children. When there is tension in the parts of the body controlled by this chakra, it reflects tension in the consciousness, an attachment or an aversion, concerning food or sex, or having children, or all of these. It may also reflect suppressed emotions about something that happened in the person's life at the time the symptom appeared.

Element: The element associated with the Orange Chakra is water. The Orange Chakra, then, reflects the individual's relationship with water. If there is a non-harmonious relationship with water (with swimming, or with being on a boat, for example), the individual's relationship with water will reflect the relationship with the parts of consciousness that water represents, that is, food and sex.

When there is a symptom that results in the person's inability to have children, we say that it begins with a decision made to not have children. This is because everything begins in our own consciousness, and the body carries out the decisions of the consciousness. Since we believe that anything can be healed, it is possible to reverse old decisions by acknowledging them, and make new ones, at deep levels of being, and then watch the body carry out these new decisions.

This chakra represents the communication between the body and the consciousness residing within. The body communicates what it wants, and what it needs. Its needs are communicated through appetite, so that if the body needs potassium, for example, on the physical level, it will communicate through the appetite a taste for a banana, or for another food containing potassium, and for as much of this food as the body needs. The inner being within the body can respond to this communication as it wishes.

The body is the vehicle for the consciousness, as an automobile is for the driver in it. If the automobile communicates through its instruments that it needs gasoline, the intelligent response is to give it what it needs, and not to decide that it should have something different.

In our society, we have learned to not trust our appetite, but rather to become more and more dependent on what experts tell us we should have. Different experts, however, have different ideas, and different activities generate different individual needs. A secretary has nutritional needs different from those of a coal miner, for example. A good relationship with the Orange Chakra includes good communication between the body and the consciousness, about what the body should have, and the honoring of that communication.

The Orange Chakra is associated with the pleasure principle. That is, we are attracted to what is pleasurable, within the areas of food and sex. The aspect of communication between the body and the consciousness, however, must always be kept in mind. For example, we may want some things for pleasure that our bodies are not interested in. After having eaten a quart of chocolate ice cream, our attachment to sensation may be telling us that we can fit in a bit more, but at the same time, our body will be telling us that it has had enough. If it has more, that will result in discomfort, rather than pleasure.

We must listen to our body, and what feels good for it. If our appetite, when we listen to it, results in discomfort within the physical body, then it is no longer serving its primary purpose of providing fuel for the physical vehicle, and we must re-establish clearer communication through releasing attachments, until we again function clearly in this part of our consciousness, and in relationship with what our bodies are asking for.

We might also consider that the appetite always works as it should, and that discomfort in the body as the result of certain eating habits just shows the parts of our consciousness and energy system that are out of balance. For example, we can ask ourselves what chakra is located at the place of the discomfort, and see that as a part of our consciousness that had not been clear. In any event, pain or discomfort is a signal that something is out of balance and needs to change, so that we can return to our natural state of harmony.

In the same way as our appetites work, our bodies respond sexually to some things and not to others. If we listen to our bodies, they tell us what is pleasurable for us, free of imposed moralities or other people's ideas of what is right. Here, we are concerned only with the question of what works for us, and what does not.

If there is some symptom that affects our sexual functioning, it is a clear signal that some things we have been doing, or some attitudes we have been holding, have not been working for us, and need to change.

Within the Body Mirror System, we make a distinction between love and sex. They are different parts of our energy system, and it is we who decide whether or not we choose to combine them, and how. The Orange Chakra represents our relationship with the pleasure we receive from our own physical body. It is concerned, then, with pure sensation, and what it feels, and not with our ideas of what it *should* feel.

When there is a symptom on one side of the Orange Chakra or the other, we can see which tension in the consciousness that symptom represents, by considering the Orange Chakra in its aspect of communication from the body to the consciousness. For example, a problem with the will ovary (the ovary on the will side) represents tension in the woman's consciousness in the area of sexuality (because the ovaries control sexuality), concerning conflict (tension is conflict) between what her body is asking for, and her will. The body is saying, "I want that," and her will is saying, "I don't want you to want that."

If the tension were on the emotional side, then we would interpret that as a conflict between what the body is asking for and the emotions. It should be emphasized here that the problem is not about what we allow ourselves to do or not do, but rather what we will allow ourselves to feel and acknowledge as what is true for us.

When our primary motivating force in life is sensation, the pleasure we receive from our body, we can say that our Orange Chakra is our home during that part of our life. From that chakra, we move our consciousness to other chakras, depending on where we choose to put our attention in any moment.

While the Orange Chakra is concerned with our relationship with food and sex, there are some symptoms involving food and sex that are not really related to this chakra. For example, bulimia is an eating disorder in which someone has an appetite, but is not receiving nourishment from the food they are eating. The chakras causing the problem are actually the Red Chakra, which has to do with the willingness of the person to be nourished, and the Yellow Chakra, which is rejecting the nourishment, through vomiting. Tensions in that chakra can be related to extreme sensitivity about freedom.

Someone with a severely blocked Red Chakra may not function well sexually, but be without any problems in the Orange Chakra. While the ovaries, for example, are controlled by the Orange Chakra, the lips to the vagina are controlled by the Red Chakra. The corresponding process in men involves the prostate gland being controlled by the Red Chakra, while the testes, and therefore the sexual drive, is controlled by the Orange Chakra.

Those experiencing a lot of insecurity may not function well sexually, but this will change when the Red Chakra is healed. It is for this reason that within some systems, the Red Chakra is mistakenly seen as the sexual chakra. A map of the nerves will show that the gonads are controlled by the lumbar plexus, associated with the Orange Chakra, and not the sacral plexus, which is associated with the Red Chakra.

While the Green Chakra, the Heart Chakra, is associated with the relational aspects of the sense of touch, it is the Orange Chakra which is involved in the aspect of touch having to do with sensation and feeling on the physical and emotional levels, as a communication from the physical body to the consciousness inside it. The Orange Chakra is concerned primarily with our own experience of what is pleasurable, and what is not. It is concerned with the pleasure that we feel from our own body.

In terms of the various bodies, the Orange Chakra is associated with the emotional body, and with our willingness to feel our emotions. The emotions that we feel will be related to and depend upon which other chakras are involved, but what we are speaking of here is the general process of allowing ourselves to feel. For example, we can listen very mechanically to music that we hear, or we can allow ourselves to be moved by the music, to feel it. This decision to feel it, in general, is associated with the Orange Chakra, while what it is that we feel will depend upon the content of the music, and the key in which it is played.

If we have had an experience that generates very strong emotions that are difficult for us to face, for example, a sense of betrayal by someone who had been very close and trusted, this may be so traumatic for us that we may decide at a deep level to not feel the resistances that are so traumatic for us. One woman, who had a particularly difficult emotional experience with her former son-in-law, afterward experienced a sense of frigidity, not letting herself feel the messages from her body with regard to sex with her husband. She had turned off all aspects of the Orange Chakra.

Thus, someone experiencing symptoms that point to tensions in their Orange Chakra, and in the parts of consciousness that this chakra represents, can look at the relationship that exists among all of these aspects. For example, we can examine the similarities in our relationships with food, sex, and our emotions.

It may be discovered that these relationships all mirror each other, or that one is emphasized while another is minimized. For example, if sexual satisfaction is suppressed, appetite for food may be increased. The person has thus chosen a different way to satisfy the desires of the Orange Chakra. If more food is put into the body than the Orange Chakra is asking for, this chakra may turn itself off, so that the desire for sex is affected.

Looking at ourselves in this way, we can see what we need to do in order to return to the experience that we know to be our individual state of balance and wholeness. Over- and under-activities can be balanced again, and we can decide to do whatever is necessary in order to return to our natural state of harmony.

We know that *anything can be healed.*

The Yellow Chakra

Also known as: Solar Plexus Chakra, Power Center, *Manipura.*

Location: Solar Plexus.

Parts of the body: The parts of the body associated with this chakra include the muscular system, the skin as a system, the solar plexus, the large intestine, stomach, liver, and other organs and glands in the region of the solar plexus.

In the endocrine system, the pancreas is the gland associated with this chakra.

Sense: The physical sense associated with this chakra is the sense of sight. Therefore, the organs of sight, the eyes, are also associated with the Yellow Chakra.

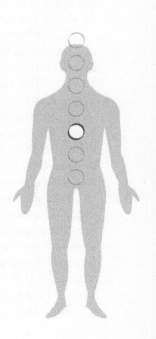

Consciousness: Parts of the consciousness associated with this chakra include perceptions concerned with power, control, freedom, the ease with which we are able to be ourselves—ease of being. Mental activity is also associated with this chakra.

Since the Yellow Chakra is associated with the sense of sight, everyone with impaired vision can be said to experience tension in their consciousness about the aspects of consciousness associated with this chakra. The nature of our physical sight is a reflection of our way of being. Nearsighted people see what is close to them easier than they see what is far away. Their direction of attention is toward the inside, or away from the outside. Their response to a threatening world is to retreat inward, and they see the world through a perceptual filter of insecurity or fear. There is tension not only in their Yellow Chakra, but also in their Red Chakra.

Farsighted people see what is farther away, rather than what is close to them. Their direction of attention is away from the inside, expanding, holding away the outside. Their response to a threatening world is to hold it away, and they see the world through a perceptual filter of anger or guilt. There is tension not only in their Yellow Chakra, but also in their Blue Chakra.

People who have astigmatism have a distorted view of what they want or what they feel, depending on whether the will eye, or the spirit eye (the emotional eye) is affected. They decide that what they really want or really feel is inappropriate for some reason, and they decide what it should be instead, believing that which they decided, rather than what was real for them. Their vision shows them that theirs is a distorted view. Other chakras besides the Yellow Chakra are affected, and which ones are affected depends upon which perceptions are being distorted. Inability to see, from the point of view that the person has created it, can be described as an unwillingness to see something. Any symptom that affects our vision, therefore, can be described as beginning with an unwillingness to see something, or with not wanting to look at some issue in our life about which we are unhappy. If we would be willing to look at it and see how we feel about it, we would have to resolve to do something about it.

Color blindness describes the person's relationship with various chakras. For example, an inability to tell the difference between red and green can be seen as reflecting an inability to tell the difference between security and love, the aspects of the Red Chakra and Green Chakra, respectively. When this is cleared, proper perceptions of colors can be restored.

In the endocrine system, when the pancreas is affected (as with diabetes), the symptom is described as an inability to tolerate sugar. Described from the point of view that the individual has created it, we would say instead that they are keeping sweetness away from themselves. When someone gets too close with sweetness, they feel threatened in their power to be themselves, and an emotion comes up, designed to create a safe distance. The emotion is anger. Diabetes is therefore associated with suppressed anger, and comes about at a time in someone's life when they are angry about something, but do not feel the freedom to express the anger. Since the pancreas is on the feeling or emotional side of the Yellow Chakra, we can see it as tension or conflict between the person's emotions and their ease of being. It is an emotional reaction. If it were on the will side, we would be able to see it as a conflict with their will.

Diabetes is considered a hereditary disease, but we can also choose to see any illness as associated with a particular way of being. If, in a family, a child imitates a way of being that has predisposed a parent to a particular symptom, the child can create the same symptom in itself. When that way of being is changed, the symptom can be released.

While diabetes can be seen as representing a rejection of sweetness, hypoglycemia represents the opposite. The person is soliciting sweetness, or expressions of love, through a pretended weakness and perceived helplessness. Symptoms in other organs associated with this chakra (liver, gall bladder, spleen) are also associated with unsuccessful ways of dealing with anger.

Element: The element associated with the Yellow Chakra is fire, and the relationship we have with fire, or the sun, can be seen to have its parallels in our relationship with the parts of the consciousness that this chakra represents. Someone sensitive about the sun, then, can be seen to have particular sensitivities about power, or control, or freedom. If there is a skin condition that makes it appear that the person has had too much sun, we can interpret it as excessive energy or attention at the level of the solar plexus chakra.

When our primary motivating force in life is freedom or power, we can say that our Yellow Chakra is our home during that part of our life.

The Yellow Chakra is also associated with the mental body, and therefore, with the activity of the mind. Those with excessive activity in the mind also experience tension in the Yellow Chakra.

The mind is a tool of the consciousness, and only a part of the consciousness. Obviously, there are other parts, for example, the soul, and the spirit.

When a child comes into the world, it is a soul manifesting through an individualized consciousness, the spirit. It also has a mind, associated with the Yellow Chakra, which it uses to learn. It is rewarded with love for learning things like responding to certain sounds (its name), and for behaving in certain ways. It soon begins to identify itself in terms of what it knows, rather than who it is, and develops what we call the personality, also at the level of the Yellow Chakra. This personality, then, is its identification with its mind, and this level of being has been defined in our Western society as the societal norm, our definition of "normal."

Sometimes the personality is in accord with the spirit, and sometimes it seems to be pulling in another direction, creating tension, until the two can be aligned. The inner being or higher self, the spirit, may want something, while the personality can have difficulty with that, living with society-based inhibitions. Some of these inhibitions can be valuable, protecting society, but others only serve to keep people from being themselves, and from living their truth. Tensions thus created can eventually create symptoms, until we return to who we really are, and live that, choosing to no longer be at the effect of self-limiting ideas. We can also then choose to live in those parts of society that value those ways of being which make us happy, and which are natural for us.

Because of this identification with mental activity, many people in our Western society do not feel comfortable with allowing the mind to rest, even though they would like to experience inner peace. The mind has stopped being just a tool, and has become the master.

To restore mastery over the mind is to consciously decide which thoughts to accept or reject, choosing perceptions rather than being at their effect, and being able to allow the mind to rest in inactivity until it is needed for analytical processes. In this way, there is increased ability to be present and see things as they are, rather than through a perceptual filter of our ideas of what is true. There is also more peace and quiet in our consciousness, and an increased ability to communicate with other levels of our consciousness, rather than negating intuitive impulses with ideas, and with reasons to not follow these impulses.

When the personality pulls in a direction different from the spirit, it is often called the ego. While many spiritual disciplines are oriented toward destroying or subjugating the ego, we can also see this as a way of fighting with a part of ourselves, creating additional tensions by discriminating against that part of us, and thus making it more difficult for us to free ourselves from the process.

What makes more sense is an acceptance of every part of ourselves, combined with a conscious choice to align ourselves with what is true for us at deep levels, aligning the personality and the spirit, and thus removing the tension without having to diminish or destroy any part of who we are.

One way to do this is by deciding that what has happened in our lives has been what we have really wanted to happen, reflecting deep decisions we have made. When we recognize this, we acknowledge that Spirit has been guiding us, and we are able to release tensions about the past, placing ourselves in the present, and re-orienting ourselves more positively toward the future.

We can also decide that we have been doing the right thing in some way, even though we may not have been aware of the good reason for our actions. They have been in keeping with our values and our sensitivities, which are the bases of our priorities and all our decisions.

This is in keeping with the Tibetan philosophy that states that because of who we are, and always have been, and always will be, there is never a need to apologize for or excuse ourselves for our actions. From that point of view, each of us has always been guided by spirit, always doing the right thing, according to the values by which we live.

We can, of course, also choose to recognize certain past ways of being that have not been working for us, regardless of the justification we created for those ways of being, and then decide that we no longer have to do things that way. We can recognize different priorities, establish different values on the bases of these priorities, and therefore we can have another experience of ourselves. In that moment, we allow another way of being that works better for us to occur in our consciousness, and we experience more peace within ourselves.

We do not have to continue to identify with or justify the actions of the being that no longer exists. Rather, we can see that being with compassion, and get on with the rest of our new life. We release ourselves from our self-imposed suffering, and are re-born in that moment into another experience of being that feels much better, and in which we can experience much more happiness. Then, we are also able to experience the freedom in our consciousness to explore deeper levels of being that are considered more evolved.

In some healings, if the subject experiences some nausea, it shows that while the deep part of the person has asked for and received a healing, there is still some holding on at the level of the personality, with the associated tensions at the level of the solar plexus. Reaffirming the decision to accept the healing that is wanted at deep levels, and the changes in consciousness that necessarily accompany the healing, serve to greatly ease the process, making it much more gentle.

This also illustrates the process of aligning the personality, the ego, with decisions made at deep levels of consciousness, at the level of the spirit, so that the whole being and all of its parts is aligned in common intention. The personality has a chance to agree with the decision that it knows to be a true reflection of what the entire being wants deeply, and what it knows to be good for itself. The personality has then aligned its intention with the spirit and the soul, and discovers a new sense of cooperation with them.

In summary, always do what you really want to do, deeply. Do not do what you really do not want to do, deeply. Throughout it all, always be who you really are, and trust your trip. If you have forgotten this basic rule of life, and have gone out of balance, you can be reassured by reminding yourself of your inner truth, that you are here to be happy, and that *anything can be healed.*

The Green Chakra

Also known as: Heart Chakra, Living Love Center, *Anahata*.

Location: Center of the chest.

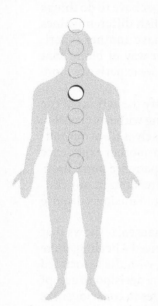

Parts of the body: This chakra is associated with the heart and circulatory system, and the cardiac plexus, as well as the lungs and the entire chest area. The endocrine gland associated with this chakra is the thymus, which controls the immune system.

Sense: The physical sense associated with this chakra is the sense of touch. This sense (touch) can be related to the Orange Chakra in its aspect of sensation, but here it is in relation to how we feel about being touched, and about the aspect of relating to the consciousness within the body.

Note: With those who are sensitive about being touched, we consider it as related to what is happening in their Green Chakra. Similarly, people who like to touch others as they speak are relating from their Green Chakra as they communicate. Those who experience insensitivity in a particular part of their body or on their skin, or numbness, would be said to be keeping themselves from feeling, which would relate more to the Orange Chakra, in its role of willingness to feel, as with emotions.

When someone is receiving a massage, it can be a purely physical experience, like being treated as a piece of steak, with purely physical manipulation, or the masseur can have sensitivity to the individual inside the body, having a sense of what that person is experiencing being touched in that way, and modifying techniques on the basis of relating to consciousness inside the body. When such relating is there, it is the sense of touch that we associate with the Heart Chakra.

Consciousness: All of the previous chakras were involved with our experience within ourselves and about ourselves, but beginning with the Green Chakra, we are involved with our relationship with the environment. The key word is "relating."

The Green Chakra is involved with relating, the area of relationships in our lives, and with our perceptions of love. In terms of relationships, it can be about partnerships, or about relating with anyone close to our heart, such as parents, or children, or siblings. When it is about loving or perceptions of being loved, it may be perceived as a process of giving or receiving love. It can also be experienced as being in a shared space in which the love is felt, and just flows, with a sense of inclusion, and not necessarily a sense of giving or receiving.

Element: The element associated with this chakra is air, and we can say that our relationship with air reflects our relationship with love. In individuals who have a problem with air, with breathing, such as asthma or emphysema, their "inability" to breathe in or out reflects their decisions about letting love in or out.

Since the thymus gland, associated with the Green Chakra, controls the immune system, those whose immune systems are affected (AIDS or HIV Positive) have a way of being that affects their perceptions of love. They perceive that their lifestyle separates them from people they love. The details of their lifestyles may differ: they may have different sexual preferences or use socially unacceptable drugs. Separation may also be due to living in a repressive society, such as that which existed in Haiti under Duvalier at the time that AIDS was born there, when members of a family did not trust others in the same family. The constant factor, though, creating AIDS, was in the person's perceptions of love, and feeling loved.

Obviously, heart problems or circulatory problems, or any symptom that affects the entire blood circulatory system can be traced to tensions in the Green Chakra and in the person's perceptions of love, and its flow.

Other symptoms that reflect tensions in the Green Chakra are those which appear in the chest or back, at the level of this chakra. Breast cancer, or other tumors or skin problems in the area of the Green Chakra are examples.

Cancer is a metaphor for things held in and not expressed, and the part of the body affected shows what was held in and not expressed. When the breast of a woman is affected, we can say that it represents something concerning her feelings about being a woman or about being a mother.

If we follow the possible logical conclusion of the illness, we can see the possibility of the breast being removed. Described from the point of view that the woman has created it herself, we would say that she has been cutting herself off from her femininity, and manifesting more masculine characteristics than is her natural state of balance. The reason for her hardness is pretty clear. She needs to get something off her chest, some resentment she has been holding in the area of the Green Chakra, in the area of relating and relationships. She feels bad about something that has happened, and has made a decision that she does not want to live with the situation any longer.

If the symptom is on the feeling or emotional side of the Green Chakra, we can say that there is a conflict involving emotions within a relationship, and if on the will side, a conflict involving the will, or what the person wants. We can also look at the symptom from the point of view of the masculine and feminine sides of the body, and ask whether it makes sense to see it as a conflict with a man or with a woman.

The same symptoms can affect a man, but this is far less common. When it does happen, the meaning is the same, regarding the individual's balance between those characteristics we define as masculine, and those we define as feminine.

When the Green Chakra needs to open more, it may be simply a process of evolution, where individuals have made the decision that they would like to experience more love than the traditionally accepted definitions of love have allowed, or where they have decided to move the home of their consciousness to the Green Chakra.

It may also be a need dictated by the necessity to heal some symptom that has been clearly related to our perceptions of love, or of its lack, when resentments, judgments, and expectations have been allowed to get in the way of these perceptions of love. Any reason we may have for closing the door to love, or to not feel love, is not a good enough reason.

With the association that the Green Chakra has with the immune system, we can recognize the importance of love in our lives. We can see that it is necessary for our survival, and that without this love, people decide that they would prefer to not live.

When the Heart Chakra, the Green Chakra, has been closed, acceptance can be used as a key, as a point of reference, for the opening process. The word can have different meanings, depending on how it is seen through our filter of perceptions, our bubble. Thus, it can be related to the individual perceptions that must change for us to experience more of the love that is available to us, through the way we can choose to see things.

Healing begins with an emotional acceptance that there is something that needs to be healed. Otherwise, there is so much denial that the resistance to the situation takes away the attention and energy that is directed to the healing.

Acceptance that something needs to be healed allows the act of self-love of wanting the healing to happen.

Acceptance of the healing allows the acceptance of the state of consciousness in which the symptom is released, and no longer exists. It can also be used as a reminder that the love surrounding the person needs to be accepted by them, in order for it to have the healing effect for which it is known.

The opening of the Green Chakra can be a process of self-acceptance, replacing self-judgment with self-love. Rather than giving ourselves reasons to believe that we must change our natural way of being and what is true for us in some way, we can realize the importance of accepting our individuality and our uniqueness. We can each acknowledge the way of being that is natural for us, not judging that way of being, and then see how it is appreciated by others.

We can then choose to spend more time with those who appreciate and love us as we are. With this self-acceptance comes an acceptance of other people's individuality and the sense of appreciation that accompanies it. As others are accepted for who they are, and their way of being is no longer judged, appreciation of who that being is has the space to grow in us, and we feel better for that.

When there are no expectations, others are not expected to change any part of their being that is natural for them. They can be seen as they are in the moment of experience. This removal of judgments and expectations from our perceptions leaves us with a good feeling, experienced in the heart, and this, we know, is acceptance, also known as love. When we have our perceptions at the level of the Green Chakra, it seems as we look around ourselves that the entire world is functioning from that space. It seems that everyone's actions have love as their basic motivating force. It looks like everyone is motivated by love, and sometimes reacting to the perception that it is not there, because different people have learned different ways of expressing the love that they feel.

One person may express love by telling others what to do, because when that was done to them, they understood it to be an expression of love. Obviously, for others, this can be understood in another way, because they may feel that someone who really loves them would not want to control their lives by telling them how to behave or what to do; instead, they would rather acknowledge their ability to make their own decisions and be the fullest expression of who they can be.

In this area, for example, parents express their love by parenting, but children become adults and may no longer want to be parented. If the children (now grown) reject that expression of the parents' love, the parents try harder, and can easily perceive that their children no longer love them. The child says, "If my parents really loved me, they would not tell me what to do. Since they are telling me what to do, they do not accept me as I am." The parents say, "My child no longer listens to me, so doesn't love me any more."

It's important to look beyond the expression of love to the feeling behind it, so that the perception of love remains. For example, an adult (son or daughter) can tell their parents, "Thanks for wanting to help me, but I want to do it my own way. I know that you love me, and that what you want for me is to be happy. Doing it my way is what will make me happy. Thank you for your love. I love you, too."

With the perception that the love is there, the tensions accompanying the misperceptions of its absence can be released. Without these tensions, and the symptoms that had accompanied them, we can again perceive the world around us in another way that works better for us, and in which we are healed.

Love heals.

Anything can be healed.

The Blue Chakra

Also known as: Throat Chakra, Cornucopia Center, *Visuddha.*

Location: Base of the throat.

Parts of the body: This chakra controls, on the physical level, the throat and neck, and the arms and hands, and is associated with the brachial or cervical plexus.

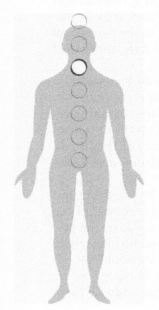

The endocrine gland associated with this chakra is the thyroid.

Sense: The physical sense associated with this chakra is the sense of hearing and, therefore, also the organs of the sense of hearing, the ears.

Consciousness: The Blue Chakra is associated with the aspects of expressing and receiving, as well as beliefs concerning the manifestation of our goals. It is also associated with the process of listening to our intuition, as well as the state of consciousness we experience when we flow with that process. Some call it abundance, while others know it as grace.

This is also the first level of consciousness from which we experience directly a sense of interaction with what some call Higher Intelligence, and with our relationship with the space around us, our space.

Element: The element associated with this chakra is known as the ether, which is defined as the most subtle physical element, corresponding on the physical level to deep space. It is an emptiness, to be sure, a void, but one that is still considered part of the physical universe.

In terms of the process of expression that we associate with the Blue Chakra, this can represent communication and discussion. It can also represent the expression of what is true for us, or expressing what is within. In this sense, it also refers to various forms of expression, such as dancing, playing music, painting, or any other process designed to bring out something that is within, when it is done as the primary purpose of that activity, doing it for its own sake, to express something.

The Blue Chakra, in its aspect of receiving, controls the arms and hands, which represent, respectively, reaching for and having. If someone injures their arm, for example, and therefore is not able to reach out, when we describe the symptom from the point of view of the person having created it, we would say that they are keeping themselves from reaching for something. That means that they have been giving themselves reasons for not going for their goals. They have been holding themselves back, and giving themselves reasons for not believing they can achieve their goals.

If the will arm was affected, they have been keeping themselves from going for what they want, and if it was the feeling, or emotional, arm, they have been keeping themselves from going for what will make them happy. We function optimally when what we want is also what will make us happy.

If it is the throat which is affected on the will side, they have felt resistance to expressing what they want, and if the feeling side, resistance to expressing their feelings. In the sense of expressing what we want in order to have what we want, or expressing our feelings in order to have what makes us happy, the Blue Chakra reflects the biblical statement, "Ask, and it shall be given you; seek, and you shall find; knock, and it shall be opened unto you."

The state of consciousness at the level of the Blue Chakra is associated with abundance, which is obviously related to the degree to which we allow ourselves to receive. The Blue Chakra, as previously mentioned, is associated with listening to our intuition, which we are told leads us successfully to the accomplishment of our goals. We are told that we can trust it, always. It comes from the deepest part of our inner being, from the place where all is known, from Universal Consciousness, and is customized for us through our individualized consciousness, our spirit. It respects our goals and our sensitivities, so that we can allow ourselves to be guided toward what we want, and away from those situations that are sensitive for us or to which we feel resistance.

When we listen to our intuition, we follow an effortless flow, moving with things that have a tendency to happen, and accepting, without resisting, the tendency that some things have to not happen. We continue being ourselves, and also acknowledge what is true for us in every moment. Obviously, if our intuition is guiding us within the present moment, it relates only to what is going on in the present moment, and to the decisions we need to make in the present moment.

When we flow in this way, things happen in a certain way that creates a perception that life provides all of our needs with no effort on our part at all. We think of things, and they happen. It is a flowing state of being in which things manifest.

It's a magic space, considered by some to be a mystical state of consciousness, because of the direct perception of interacting with another level of consciousness that some people call God. Others may call this consciousness Holy Spirit, or The Universe, or Superconscious, or Higher Intelligence. The important aspect of the perception is not the name, but rather the sense of interaction with another level of being.

Some describe this state of consciousness as grace, where it seems to the individual that everything they want for themselves, God also wants for them and delivers it. From this state of consciousness, it can seem as though the Universe is a benevolent entity, and that seemingly unrelated events have a pattern and order to them, existing as a conspiracy to make the individual happy. Some describe it as a positive paranoia.

Others may personify the benevolent entity they perceive. Jesus personified it as the Father. Thus, He could say, "It is not I who does these things, but My Father." It was evident to Jesus that what was happening was beyond what He was doing on a personal level, and that another level of intelligence was working with Him. This is the view from the Blue Chakra.

The Blue Chakra can function in this state of grace or abundance either alone, or in combination with the Green Chakra.

When the Blue Chakra is functioning in combination with the Green Chakra, then what the Universe provides comes through an expression of love. You follow your flow, filled with love, and expressing your love, and in that way, providing others' needs with no effort on their part, and so your needs are met in the same way, which is through an expression of love. Doing nice things for others because you really want to encourage others to want to do nice things for you, as well. Do unto others as you would have others do unto you.

The key to remaining in this space is for us to continue to flow in the expression of our love, and to acknowledge and appreciate that which is received as being the answer to what had been asked for, in consciousness. It was a gift from Spirit, delivered through the individual who was moved to function in that way through the expression of *their* love.

Concerning the association of the element of ether with the Blue Chakra, within our model of the physical universe as defined with the chakras, we have reached the subtlest physical element. However, we have two more chakras that we have not yet discussed. The elements associated with the next two chakras, then, must be non-physical elements, or spiritual elements, not existing in the physical universe.

Within this model, we can say that what we know as the physical universe is projected onto another dimension, the one we call spiritual. From the spiritual point of view, we define the ether as the matrix upon which the physical universe is projected. It is the place where thought forms exist as holographic images, and onto these three-dimensional thought forms, the physical elements are projected, to achieve full manifestation in the physical universe.

The ether, then, can also be seen as the crossover between the physical and spiritual universes. When the consciousness of the individual is in this place, the state of grace previously described is being experienced.

There is a relationship that exists between the Red Chakra and the Blue Chakra. While the Red Chakra can be said to represent our beliefs about having our needs met, the Blue Chakra is about having our "wants" met. If we don't have much of a belief in having our survival needs met, it may be difficult for us to believe in the sense of abundance that the Blue Chakra represents. This can be reflected in our relationship with money.

With the Red Chakra, money represents security. With the Blue Chakra, money represents a reward from the Universe for a job well done. We do an activity for the sake of doing it, enjoying what we do, and the Universe supports us in that. We accept this support by allowing ourselves to be paid for what we do, even though that was not our primary reason for doing that thing. Or, we can allow ourselves to receive something in exchange for what we do, being comfortable with the process.

At the level of the Blue Chakra, then, we decide the lifestyle in which we choose to live, and notice that the Universe supports us in that lifestyle. We just continue to do what we really want to do, and not do what we really do not want to do, and notice that our needs are always met in the moment, with no effort on our part at all. As we think of things, these things happen. Then, we are experiencing abundance, and life in the Blue Chakra.

Remarkable healings happen in this space.

Anything can be healed.

The Indigo Chakra

Also known as: Brow Chakra, Consciousness, Awareness Center, Third Eye, *Ajna.*

Location: Center of the forehead.

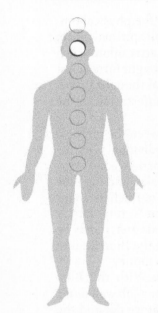

Parts of the body: This chakra is associated with the forehead and temples, with the carotid plexus, and with the pituitary gland, the master controller of the endocrine system. Dysfunction of this chakra is associated with problems of physical growth, creating gigantism or dwarfism.

Sense: The sense associated with the Indigo Chakra is the set of all inner senses that correspond to each of the outer physical senses. For example, the outer sense of eyesight is associated with clairvoyance, the outer sense of hearing is associated with the inner sense of clairaudience, and so on. The combination of all these inner senses is known as Extra Sensory Perception, or ESP, the set of senses beyond the physical. It is spirit-to-spirit communication. Our natural abilities to communicate with Spirit or spirits, to feel and see subtle energies, and to work with them, are associated with this chakra.

Consciousness: This chakra is associated with the deep inner level of being we call spirit, the place where our true motivations are found, which Western society knows as the subconscious, or unconscious. It is also associated with what we consider spirituality, and the spiritual perspective.

Element: The element associated with this chakra is a vibration, a nonphysical element, known as the inner sound. It is the sound which we hear in our ears which does not depend upon a source in the physical world. While our Western society considers it a pathological condition whose cause is not known, the ability to hear it is considered within some of the Eastern traditions (Kriya Yoga, for example, into which I was initiated) as a prerequisite to further spiritual growth.

Within some of these traditions, there is actually an entire set of inner sounds, each one of which has a particular meaning, communicating to us something about what is happening in our experience at that time. It may be a transcendent experience accompanied by the cosmic music, that music which to some sounds like angels singing or that which inspired musicians like Mozart.

It may also be a sound of the intensity of energy during a process of transformation, of movement between two paradigms. It may also be experienced as a whistle, or a rushing sound, or a ringing. Most commonly, when it is experienced as a problem, it is the deeper aspect of our spirit, catching our attention like an alarm clock, and asking us to examine what is true for us at deep levels, when we have not been paying attention to that, and not listening to ourselves.

One woman from the United States, for example, was visiting her daughter in Europe, and when it was time for her to return home, because she thought she should, a ringing began in her ears. Her inner being, which she had not been listening to at the time, wanted to catch her attention and ask her what she really wanted to do. In fact, she really wanted to stay in Europe, and when she made that decision, the ringing in her ears stopped.

Thus, we can see the association of this chakra with deeper parts of our consciousness, from the level called spirit, or the spiritual, and with seeing what is true for us at that level, since it is that which is actually directing our lives.

From this level of perception, we can each observe our actions, our outer theater, from the place of knowing in that moment what our motivations are behind these actions, our inner theater. We can see when our actions are those that are designed to have a particular effect or to solicit a particular response.

The Indigo Chakra can also represent our relationship with our philosophical, spiritual, or religious views, since it is these that are intended to give us an understanding of this level of our being. The details of these spiritual views are not important here, but just the question of whether or not we are in harmony with them.

From a spiritual perspective associated with the Indigo Chakra, we can see that we attract to ourselves those experiences that reflect our desires, our fears, and our beliefs, the pictures we put into our consciousness, and we can see that others do the same. We can see that all of the events in our lives reflect the decisions we have made, whether or not we remember those decisions when the events happen. Our decisions create events in the outer world that move in a way to carry out those decisions.

Since we each create our own reality, we can see the amazing interactions we create with other creators. It is as though we are the main character in our own movie, with all of our friends playing their favorite roles in support of ours, and at the same time, we are playing supporting roles for each of our friends, who are the main characters in their movies.

This complex interaction functions perfectly, according to that which we each create and agree to play. When we see healing as a process of co-creation, we are seeing it from the point of view of this chakra, and we can see that what happens during the healing is a function of what each of us brings to it.

It is as if we are each a dreamer dreaming a dream, and projecting our dream around ourselves, like a bubble. In considering ourselves as creators, we can acknowledge that each of us, and all of us, are creators, projecting our respective bubbles. Where these bubbles interpenetrate each other, we co-create a three-dimensional hologram, which we agree to call external physical reality. The events in this external physical world, then, reflect what was happening in the consciousness of the individuals involved in that event.

Since it is from this place that we create events in the physical world, we are able to work in ways that seem to override physical laws, or create sequences of amazing physical events, which carry out the decisions we have made, regarding the healing. Biological structure changes in accordance with and as the effect of our perceptions.

When we see the co-creation of the healing from this point of view, we are also able to see other events in our lives in the same way, giving us additional levels of understanding, as well as the means for stepping beyond other self-imposed limits, and truly seeing ourselves as creators.

Working with this chakra, we can see how the person being healed is feeling inside the physical vehicle that their body represents, how they feel about their vehicle, and what is happening for them at the level of their spirit.

During one healing, a woman remembered the experience of her birth, which was caesarian. In cutting open the mother, the doctor cut the baby, so that her first experience, before even coming into the world, was one of pain. When she was able to return to the level of consciousness that she had experienced just before that birth, she felt better about what she was on earth to do. In addition, over the next few days, she grew seven and a half centimeters (three inches), and the color of her eyes changed.

When remarkable results like these are achieved, we are able to see that we are not limited by the so-called laws of genetics, physics, chemistry or biology, and that the most powerful force in the Universe is the consciousness within each of us.

It is this consciousness within us that is who we really are, and not the vehicle, the body with which we may have identified. We are the spirit within the body, which entered the body at birth, and which leaves it after the process we call death. This being that we each are is, in fact, immortal, continuing to experience other dimensions after this lifetime is completed, in a process that lasts indefinitely.

The perceptions we have after leaving the body are those of the spiritual view, which feel much better than the petty human values to which we may have become accustomed. The place from which we experience these values is what some people call "heaven."

We do not have to leave our body in order to enjoy these evolved points of view, nor do we have to search outside of ourselves for the kingdom of heaven. As we have been reminded before, this level of perception is within each of us, as basic equipment in our energy system.

We can live it whenever we choose. For example, we can live it now. We can live in heaven on earth now, as creators learning to recognize one another, and to then be able to relate to one another as co-creators. We can help by reminding each other (and ourselves) who we really are, and healing those around us if that is needed and wanted, holding the perception that *anything can be healed.*

The Violet Chakra

Also known as: Crown Chakra, Cosmic Consciousness Center, "I Am" Center, *Sahasrara.*

Location: Top of the head.

Parts of the body: While each of the other chakras is associated with a particular plexus, this chakra is associated with the brain, and the entire nervous system. Any symptom affecting the nervous system as a whole, such as multiple sclerosis or Parkinson's disease, reflects tension in the Violet Chakra, and the parts of the consciousness associated with this chakra. The hair and nails, essentially composed of nerve tissue, are also associated with this chakra, as is the top of the head, of course.

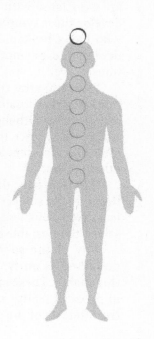

The Violet Chakra is associated with the pineal gland, most of whose functions remain a mystery to science, but which is known to be related to the production of melanin, a substance which responds to light, and which creates the pigment in our skin.

It is believed by some that when certain psychoactive substances are ingested, they do not remain in the body as such, but are converted into another substance that resembles the secretions of the pineal gland, and it is for this reason that they have their psychoactive effect. Naturally, the use of these very powerful substances is neither encouraged nor promoted here, but merely explained.

Sense: The sense associated with this chakra is empathy, which we define as experiencing another person's experience as if it were our own. It is an aspect of experiencing unity with that person.

Consciousness: The Violet Chakra represents that part of our consciousness concerned with perceptions of unity or separation. It also represents our relationship with our father, and with authority in general.

Element: The element associated with this chakra is a subtle spiritual vibration known as the inner light. It is what we experience when we are in the deepest part of our being experiencing ourselves as a single point of consciousness glowing with intelligence. This glow, although not really white and not really light, is also known as White Light, because that is the closest we can come to describing it in terms of our physical senses.

The inner light, esoterically, is considered the subtlest of the elements of which the entire physical universe is created, becoming more dense through the other elements of inner sound, ether, air, fire, water, and earth.

In the healing process, when healers enter the consciousness of the person to be healed, sometimes they feel what the subject is feeling, as if it were happening within themselves. It is easy to understand why some people believe that it is possible to take on the subject's symptoms. They may feel what the subject is feeling, in the experience we call empathy, but if healers have not created the conditions in their own consciousness that are associated with the symptom, they will not, on the physical level, develop those symptoms. If a healer is working with someone, for example, who has a broken arm or hemorrhoids, the healer obviously will not develop those symptoms. Then, the same must be true for all other symptoms, as well.

With empathy, the healer may experience not only the physical sensations, but also possibly the state of mind or the emotions, that the other is experiencing, although this is quite rare. When the symptoms are released within the subject, the healer then also experiences the release. It is a sort of feedback system letting the healer know what is happening within the other person.

If healers have this sensitivity and experience these things when they flow into the subject's consciousness, they can afterwards take off the subject's consciousness, like removing an overcoat, or flow back into themselves, to re-establish the consciousness they know to be their own.

Any of the so-called mystic states of consciousness that can be described as unity can also be said to be related to the functioning of this chakra. These may include, for example, experiencing the entire play of physical reality as a movie, a play of light and shadow, projected for the interests of the single consciousness known as the "I Am," which we each are, as a dream is projected for the interests of the dreamer. In this case, the dream appears to be outside us, but is actually just a projection of a deeper part of our consciousness. Then, everything in the dream is nothing more than an extension of our own consciousness, as the dreamer. There is then a sense of unity with all beings and all things in the dream, since they are all parts of and extensions of the same consciousness that we are.

Or, we can see ourselves as an organ within a greater organism. One person can be the ear, another the nose, another the stomach, etc., and then it would be obvious that the best way to serve the organism would be for the ear to be totally an ear, the nose totally a nose, and so on. It would not make sense for an ear to say, "I would rather be a nose."

While it is apparent that the uniqueness of each is of essential importance, it is also evident that each is connected to and part of the whole, as the fingers of a hand, while each is unique, are all connected and part of the being whose hand it is. That, too, can be seen as a sense of unity, related to the Violet Chakra, combined with the perceptions of individualized consciousness and co-creation that we associate with the Indigo Chakra.

The Violet Chakra represents the level of being we define as the soul, the deepest part of who we are. It is the part of us that travels through lifetime after lifetime. The soul takes on within a particular lifetime an individualized consciousness we call the spirit, with individualized experiences preparing us for the individualized function we have in that lifetime.

When we experience the deepest part of who we are, it can seem as if our consciousness is all that there is. We are able to experience the ultimate "I Am" consciousness. Of course, from another point of view, we know that within each and every other being, the same capability exists. They are able to experience themselves also as "I Am," all that exists.

If the deepest part of who we each are, in the deepest part of the Violet Chakra or the soul, is the same "I Am" consciousness, we are obviously ultimately all One. At this level of consciousness, we are all connected. Then, we must be aware of everything happening within everyone's consciousness. All is known, and it is for this reason that the Violet or Crown Chakra is associated with Universal Consciousness, and the Akashic Records. Western experts in consciousness also know it as the Collective Unconscious, or the Collective Subconscious.

It is from this place, then, from this level of consciosness, that intuition originates. It must, of course, come from a place where all is known in order for it to always be 100% accurate. Intuition, as previously described, is individualized for the being through the spirit. Following this intuitive voice along the path of optimal flow, or least resistance, as a free choice, is associated with the Blue Chakra.

As the Red Chakra reflected our relationship with Mother Earth, the Violet Chakra represents our relationship with Our Father (Who Art In Heaven). In the traditional family structure, the mother provides the nourishment and the safe space, and the father provides the direction. Our relationship with our biological father or father figure sets the pattern for our relationship with authority, and that sets the basis for our relationship with God, within a paradigm that includes a belief in God.

When someone experiences a sense of separation from their father, or feels not loved by him, they close the Violet Chakra. Mechanically, in terms of how the energy system functions, this creates a sense of isolation. Consequently, it is as though the person is in a shell, and it is difficult for those outside the shell to make contact with the being within, and difficult for the being within to experience contact with the outside world. They seem to be always different from those around them.

They may also experience no sense of direction, of where they are going. Their relationship with authority will reflect their attitudes towards their father, until such time as they are again able to open to their father's love, and perceive themselves as loved by their father, or by God.

Sometimes, the closing of the Violet Chakra is not a pathological process, even though it can create the same sense of isolation. It can be a spiritual process happening with someone raised within Western traditions, who has an essentially Eastern orientation.

The Western traditions present God as an authority outside ourselves, and a separation and isolation can serve the positive purpose of having us find the God within, being our own authority, and placing our belief in ourselves, yet functioning in accord with authority, and not against it. When the philosophical bases of self-belief and autonomy combined with alignment have been established, and the positive purpose of this process served, we can again open the Violet Chakra, and experience its benefits of having the choice of unity or separation, as the moment requires.

Obviously, there are times when being alone is the appropriate decision. During a meditation, for example, it may not serve us to have all of our friends and relatives galloping through our consciousness, but rather we should be re-establishing our own centeredness and tranquility, preparing us to again function with others in the world with clarity.

It is, of course, about having the choice. The choice is always ours. If we have forgotten that, we can be reminded and remembering we can be healed.

Anything can be healed.

The Language of Colors

We associate particular colors with particular chakras in a model that represents wholeness and wellness, and that we use for healing. Any other configuration of colors, then, represents something other than wellness, something that needs to be healed. There are possibilities for any other color than the natural one to be in a particular chakra, and the color that finds its way there says something particular about the condition of that chakra.

The different combinations of colors that can be found in a particular chakra represent a code, a language that everyone knows, even though they may not know that they know it. Thus, you might recognize that the language you use to describe your relationship with a certain color actually describes your relationship with the parts of your consciousness represented by the chakra with that as its natural color.

You can also recognize that when you see a color other than the natural color in a certain chakra, you are recognizing an out-of-balance condition in a way that implies knowing exactly how it is out of balance. It means that you also know exactly what needs to be done in order to return that portion of your consciousness to perfect balance. This is in accord with the idea that somewhere inside, we each know exactly where we are and what is happening inside ourselves.

In addition to the seven natural colors of the spectrum, there are other colors that may appear, which are interpreted as follows:

- **Black** means something suppressed.

- **White** means something avoided.

- **Pink** is the color of love in motion, love that is directed.

- **Gold** is the color of angels, and also the color associated with a healer healing with no personal purpose other than to see the subject healed. It's the same consciousness as angelic consciousness, which also has no personal purpose other than to serve humans.
- **Silver** is in the same octave as gold, and represents the same level of consciousness, but with a different character, in the same way that extraterrestrials give the same message as angels, but because of their different form, have access to a different portion of the population.

Any other colors or combinations of colors should be considered in terms of the combinations of the colors that they represent. For example, gray is black and white combined, brown is red and green combined, etc. The language of the colors is defined on the following pages.

Rather than focusing on the details, you are advised to get a sense of how the combinations of colors are used, and to be creative and flexible in the interpretation of the colors, in order to find the combinations of words that best speak to the individual experiencing the symptom.

Color Language Reference Guide

The Red Chakra

Any other color but red in this chakra represents what the subject sees as a "key" to security or feeling safe, or as a consideration in the area of security, something to think about in order to feel safe or feel trust. (The underlying idea is that the subject should need none of these things as a key to security, but must find it within themselves.)

- Orange in the Red: Food or sex as a key to security.
- Yellow in the Red: The mind or power, control, or freedom, as a key to security.
- Green in the Red: Relationship or love as a key to security.
- Blue in the Red: Receiving as security. Hunger for security.
- Indigo in the Red: Spirituality as a key to security.
- Violet in the Red: Unity as a key to security, or the color of the father in the place of the mother, showing the father as the nourishing energy. Confusion or reversal of sexual roles, of which attributes are considered masculine and which are considered feminine.
- Black in the Red: Suppressed fear or issues of security suppressed. Insecurity and fear regarding money, home, job, for example.
- White in the Red: Avoiding security and those issues concerned with security. Avoiding being nourished. Avoiding roots. Avoiding mother.

Red in any other chakra indicates insecurity about that chakra's attributes.

The Orange Chakra

Any other color but orange in this chakra indicates what the individual sees as a "key" to food or sex, or a consideration in that area, rather than just listening to what the body is saying.

- Red in the Orange: Insecurity about food or sex.
- Yellow in the Orange: The mind telling the body what it should have, instead of listening to the body.
- Green in the Orange: Confusion between love and sex, and interpreting sex as love. Physical attraction interpreted as love. Love as a key to sex.
- Blue in the Orange: Unfulfilled hunger for food or sex.
- Indigo in the Orange: Spirituality as a key to food or sex.
- Violet in the Orange: Unity as a key to food or sex, or the father as a consideration in the area of food or sex.
- Black in the Orange: Suppression of food or sex, or of emotions.
- White in the Orange: Avoidance of food or sex, or of emotions.

Orange in any other chakra indicates food or sex as a key to the attributes of that chakra.

The Yellow Chakra

Any other color but yellow in this chakra represents something the individual sees as a key to power, control, freedom, or self-definition.

- Red in the Yellow: Insecurity about power, control, freedom, or self-definition.
- Orange in the Yellow: Food or sex as a key to power, control, freedom, or self-definition.
- Green in the Yellow: Defining themselves in terms of their relationship, rather than what is true for themselves. In the relationship, compromising their power to be themselves. The relationship as a consideration for power, control, freedom, rather than finding it within themselves.
- Blue in the Yellow: Hunger for power, control, freedom, or self-definition.
- Indigo in the Yellow: Spirituality as a key to power, control, freedom, or self-definition.
- Violet in the Yellow: Unity as a key to power, control, freedom, or self-definition, or the father as a consideration in this area. Power issues with authority.
- Black in the Yellow: Suppressed power or anger.
- White in the Yellow: Avoidance of power. Avoiding self-definition.

Yellow in any other chakra represents the mind or power, control, or freedom as a consideration in the attributes of that chakra.

The Green Chakra

Any other color but green in this chakra indicates what the person sees as a key to relationships or love, or is a consideration in this area.

- Red in the Green: Insecurity about love or relationships.
- Orange in the Green: Confusion between love and sex. Seeing sex as a key to love. Believing no sex means no love.
- Yellow in the Green: Power, control, or freedom as a key to or consideration in relationships or love. Control issues in the relationship.
- Blue in the Green: Hunger for love or for relationships.
- Indigo in the Green: Spirituality as a key to relationships or love.
- Violet in the Green: Unity as a key to relationships or love, or the father as a consideration in this area.
- Black in the Green: Something suppressed in the area of relationships or perceptions of love.
- White in the Green: Avoiding love or relationships.

Green in any other chakra indicates relationships or love as a consideration in the attributes of that chakra.

The Blue Chakra

Any other color but blue in this chakra represents that which is considered as a key to expressing, rather than expression being natural for that which is within. Considering the Blue Chakra in its aspect of receiving, any other color but blue in this chakra represents something keeping the person from having, or a barrier to letting things in.

- Red in the Blue: Insecurity about receiving or expressing.
- Orange in the Blue: Food or sex as a key to expression, or as a preoccupation keeping the person from having.
- Yellow in the Blue: The mind and ideas keeping the person from having. Expanding energy interfering with receiving. Power or control issues interfering with receiving.
- Green in the Blue: Love or relationships as a key to expression, or love being expressed in a way that keeps the person from having it. Giving away that which is dear, as an expression of love, and depriving themselves.
- Indigo in the Blue: Spirituality as a key to expression, and keeping the person from having that which they do not consider as spiritual.
- Violet in the Blue: Unity as a key to expression, or the father (authority) as a consideration in the area of expression, and affecting the process of receiving.

- Black in the Blue: Suppressed expression of the inner being.
- White in the Blue: Avoiding expression. Avoiding communication. Avoiding having.

Blue in any other chakra indicates a hunger for that which that particular chakra represents.

The Indigo Chakra

Any other color but indigo in this chakra indicates that which the person considers as a key to spirituality.

- Red in the Indigo: Insecurity about spirituality, or identification with the physical body, rather than the spirit or consciousness in the body.
- Orange in the Indigo: Food or sex as a key to spirituality.
- Yellow in the Indigo: The mind as a key to spirituality or a mental construct of spirituality rather than direct experience. Power, control, or freedom as a consideration in the area of spirituality. Solar plexus energy in the area of spirituality.
- Green in the Indigo: Love or relationship as a key to spirituality.
- Blue in the Indigo: Hunger for spirituality.
- Violet in the Indigo: Unity as a key to spirituality, or confusion between unity and spirituality, or the father as a consideration in the area of spirituality.
- Black in the Indigo: Suppression of spirituality. Suppression of what is deeply true for the person, at the level of their spirit.
- White in the Indigo: Avoidance of spirituality. Avoiding what is deeply true for the person, at the level of their spirit.

Indigo in any other chakra indicates spirituality as a key to what that chakra represents.

The Violet Chakra

Any other color but violet in this chakra indicates that which is considered a key to unity or the father.

- Red in the Violet: Insecurity about unity, or the color of the mother in the place of the father. Confusion about masculine and feminine roles and characteristics.
- Orange in the Violet: Food or sex as a key to unity or the father.
- Yellow in the Violet: The color of power, control, or freedom in the place of the father or authority, or the mind as a key to unity.

- Green in the Violet: Love or relationship as a key to unity or the father.
- Blue in the Violet: Hunger for unity, hunger for direction, hunger for the father.
- Indigo in the Violet: Spirituality as a key to unity or the father, or confusion between unity and spirituality.
- Black in the Violet: Suppression of unity. Suppression of a deep soul experience, or of feelings regarding authority or the father, that create separation.
- White in the Violet: Avoiding unity, avoiding the father.

Violet in any other chakra indicates that unity or the father is a consideration in the part of the consciousness that the chakra represents. Violet in most or all of the other chakras shows someone searching for or seeing the father everywhere.

Using the Chakra Analysis Chart and the Healing Analysis Report

Some healers find it interesting to keep records of the healings in which they participate, in order to correlate correspondences. That is, they are able to correlate particular symptoms to particular conditions seen in the chakras.

The Chakra Analysis Chart and Healing Analysis Report shown on pages 208 and 209 are intended as examples. They can be photocopied from this book (possibly printed on reverse sides of the same sheet of paper), and used as is, or you can create your own versions, perhaps more fully adapted to your particular needs or interests.

As you work, note on the Chakra Analysis Chart what was seen while examining the subject's energy system—which colors were seen in which chakras, which thought forms were seen and removed, which conditions were seen in the roots, for example.

In cases where the healing might not be immediately total, you could compare the view of the energy system on subsequent visits of the subject, noting the stability of the healing, the degree to which the subject has accepted the changes.

On the Healing Analysis Report note the subject's name and astrological sign, the name of the symptom and its effect (how the subject experiences it), and the immediate and (possibly) delayed effects of the healing.

For the name of the symptom, you could note the medical term, for example, Asthma, and for the effects of this particular symptom, you could note, "Difficulty breathing." While this is a rather trivial and obvious example, the benefits of these separate notations would be more obvious with named symptoms that are not so familiar.

An added benefit of this separation in notation would be for rewording the effect on the subject in a way that reflects the idea that they created it (keeping themselves from breathing, in the example mentioned).

For the immediate effects of the healing, you could note all of the effects apparent at the completion of the healing (80% breathing restored, chest pain released, for example). Any additional effects becoming obvious over the period of time following the healing could be noted as delayed effects of the healing (Full breathing restored one week after healing session, for example).

It might also be interesting to see how the energy system of one subject with a particular symptom compares with the energy system of another subject with similar symptoms or to see if there is some correspondence between particular symptoms and particular astrological signs.

It is also possible then to correlate views of the energy systems of subjects having symptoms not readily identifiable in terms of their inner causes.

The Chakra Analysis Chart and the Healing Analysis Report are wonderful tools to use in order to create documentation that can also be used in professional or academic studies designed to prove that *anything can be healed.*

Chakra Analysis Chart

Name: _____ Date: _____

Colors seen

Comments (thought
forms removed)

_____

_____

_____

_____

_____

_____

_____

Earth (conditions in roots): _____

Earth (center): _____

Healing Analysis Report

Name: _____   Date: _____

M/F: _____ Birth date: _____   Astrological sign: _____

Symptoms: _____

_____

_____

_____

Effects of symptoms: _____

_____

_____

_____

Effects of healing, immediate – according to subject: _____

_____

_____

_____

Effects of healing, delayed – according to subject: _____

_____

_____

_____

Environment, comments, etc.: _____

_____

_____

_____

Signed: _____

Healing Templates

Healing with White Light

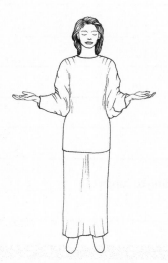

Healing Starting Position

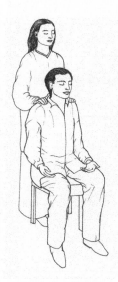

Ready to Heal

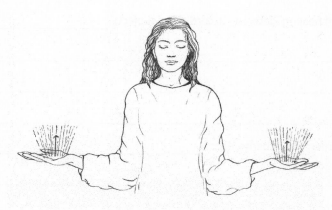

Healing Starting Position

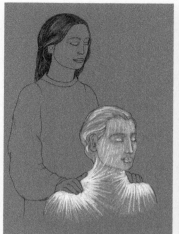
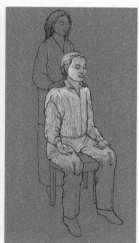

Filling the Subject

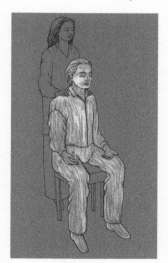

Filled with Light

Healing with Chakras and/or Thought Forms

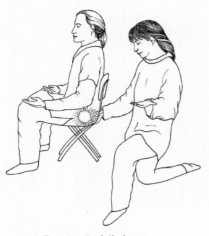

Forming Red Chakra

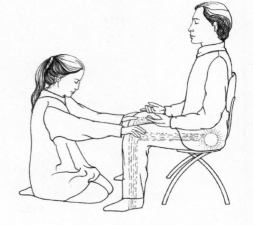

Roots to the Feet

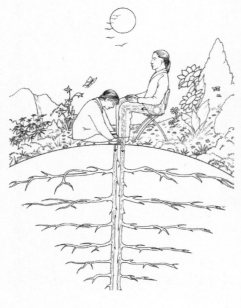

Roots in the Earth

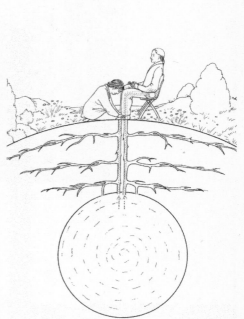

Roots Drawing in Nourishment

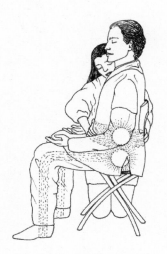

Healing the Orange Chakra

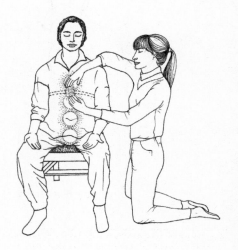

Opening the Passage

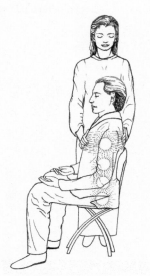

Healing the Green Chakra

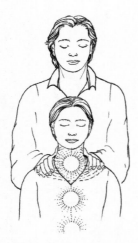

Forming the Blue Chakra

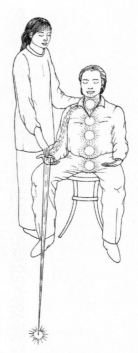

Forming Blue Laser

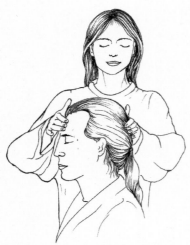

Healing the Indigo Chakra

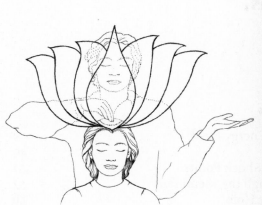

Opening the Lotus

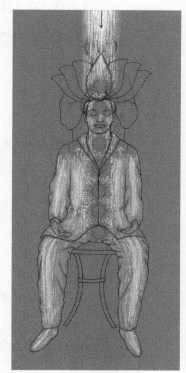

Cosmic Rinse

List of Illustrations and Exercises

Illustrations

Exercises and Meditations

Index

About the Author

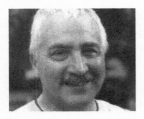

Martin Brofman dedicated his life to providing tools for healing and transformation, for self-development and spiritual awakening. He created the Body Mirror System of Healing and A Vision Workshop, as the result of his research into the body/mind connection, and from what he learned healing himself of terminal cancer in 1975. He worked with and taught these methods around the world until 2014 when he passed away.

Martin is the author of *Anything Can Be Healed, Improve Your Vision* and *The Inner Cause*, three books that have been translated into and published in more than twenty languages. As founder and director of the Brofman Foundation for the Advancement of Healing, Martin was dedicated to promoting healing in the world, as well as coordinating the activities of the various instructors teaching his methods. He believed and worked with the idea that we are all healers, and that anything can be healed. His teachings played a role in many people's lives and the quality of his love touched some very deeply.

His wife, Annick Brofman, and other instructors trained by Martin are continuing his work, teaching classes successfully around the world. The Brofman Foundation for the Advancement of Healing in Switzerland, now directed by Annick, continues to be involved in gathering information and advancing healing as a process in the world.

For information about Martin Brofman's
healing courses around the world, the Body Mirror
System and a Vision workshop, meditation and
relaxation CDs, chakra posters and more
please contact:

The Brofman Foundation for the Advancement of Healing

Annick Brofman
angel@healer.ch
+33(0)682 258 868

www.brofman-foundation.org

Also by Martin Brofman

The Inner Cause
By Martin Brofman

Exploring the body as a map of consciousness, Martin Brofman explains how physical symptoms reflect stresses on your mind, emotions, and spirit. In this book, he offers an A-to-Z compendium of 800 symptoms and a psychology of their inner causes, the messages they are trying to send to your consciousness. Informed by Brofman's long-term experience with his Body Mirror System of Healing, this compilation brings invaluable insight into how we can support the healing process.

9781844097531

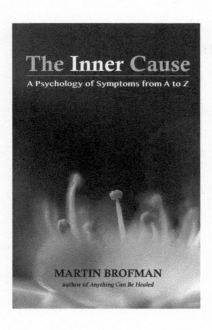

Working with Chakras for Belief Change
The Healing InSight Method
By Nikki Gresham-Record

An easy-to-use therapy tool for transforming unhelpful belief patterns and envisioning positive change, the Healing InSight Method offers a combination of chakra work, affirmations, visualization, and bodywork exercises. Unhealthy beliefs take root within the chakras and the body. A process of clearing the chakras and realigning the beliefs and their associated vibrations in the subconscious mind and energy body serves to enable any blocks to dissolve and our system to open up to the opportunity for change.

9781620559024

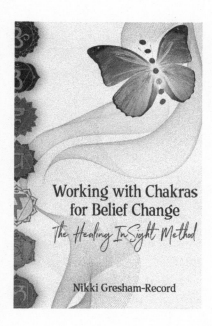

Chakra Reference Chart

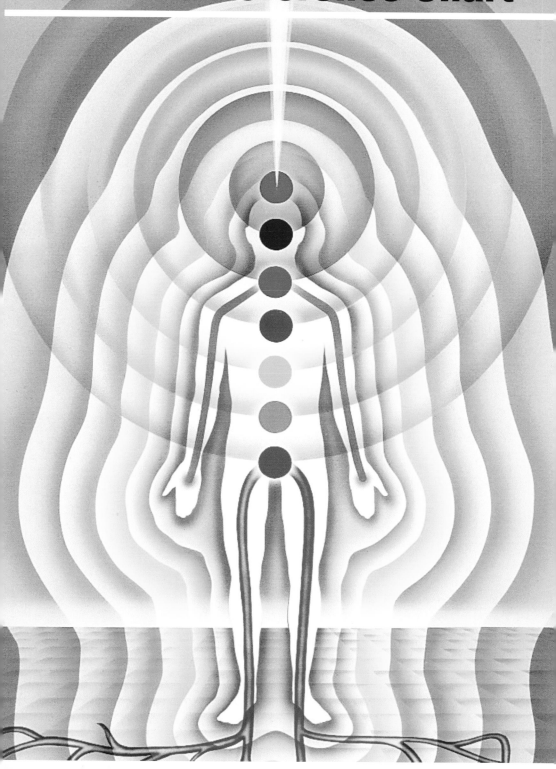

THE CHAKRAS

STRUCTURE

Yang
Male
Will
Acting

CAUSAL BODY
BUDDHIC (NIRVANIC) BODY
ETHERIC BODY
ASTRAL BODY
MENTAL BODY
EMOTIONAL BODY
PHYSICAL BODY

Vibrations	Nerves	System
Musical Notes	Glands	**Elements**
Violet	**Brain**	Nervous System
B Si	Pineal	**Inner Light**
Indigo	**Carotid Plexus**	Growth, Endocrine System
A La	Pituitary	**Inner Sound**
Blue	**Cervical Plexus**	Metabolism
G Sol	Thyroïd	**Ether**
Green	**Cardiac Plexus**	Respiration, Circulation, Immune System
F FA	Thymus	**Air**
Yellow	**Solar Plexus**	Skin, Muscles, Digestive System
E Mi	Pancreas	**Fire**
Orange	**Lombar Plexus**	Assimilation and Reproduction
D Re	Gonads	**Water**
Red	**Sacral Plexus**	Skeleton, Lymph, Elimination System
C Do	Adrenals	**Earth**

EXPERIENCE

(Deepest Inner Experience)

God
White Light
Father

CAUSAL BODY   Yin
BUDDHIC (NIRVANIC) BODY   Female
ETHERIC BODY   Spirit
ASTRAL BODY   Feeling
MENTAL BODY
EMOTIONAL BODY
PHYSICAL BODY
(Outermost Level of Experience)

Sense

Area of Consciousness

Soul   Empathy

Unity
Universal Consciousness
Source of Direction and Intuition

Spirit   Extra Sensory Perception

Spiritual Awareness
Individualized Consciousness

Hearing

Expressing, Receiving, Abundance
Flowing Manifestation
Listening to Intuition

Touch

Relating, Giving
Perceptions of Love
Acceptance

Having

Personality   Vision

Freedom/Power
Controle, Self-Definition
Intellect

Taste

Sensations
Feeling & Feelings
Food, Sex, Appetite

Smell

Safety, Security
Trust - Survival
Money, Home, Job

Mother Earth

The Body Mirror System   © 1988 Martin Brofman   Illustration and layout: Jørgen Højland

FINDHORN PRESS

Life-Changing Books

Learn more about us and our books at
www.findhornpress.com

For information on the Findhorn Foundation:
www.findhorn.org